Outcomes Assessment in End - Stage Kidney Disease - Measurements and Applications in Clinical Practice

Edited by

Paraskevi Theofilou

Sotiria Hospital for Thoracic Diseases
Athens
Greece

&

Center for Research and Technology
Department of Kinesiology
Health & Quality of Life Research Group
Trikala
Thessaly
Greece

DEDICATION

To my husband for all his support.

CONTENTS

Vereerstraeten, Guy Van Roost, Karin Caekelbergh, Mark Lamotte and Suzanne Laplante

PART VII: RESEARCH AND POLICY IMPLICATIONS

Foreword by Stanton Newman

This eBook is timely. It captures two crucial changes in health care. One is an increasing concern with the quality of patient experience. The other is a focus on the impact of treatments on patients with different types of conditions. For many years work on chronic health conditions concentrated on mortality, morbidity and symptom relief. This approach reflected an appropriate attempt by the medical profession to find a cure or better treatment for each condition. While this has remained an area of great effort, the systematic evaluation of medical interventions and treatments from the patients' perspective is now seen to be of critical importance too. There is growing recognition that patients and their family members with support and advice from healthcare professionals essentially manage most chronic conditions. Patients make decisions on what is important to them and how their treatments fit in with other aspects of their lives. This includes whether they should follow all the medical advice and adhere absolutely to treatments.

In end - stage kidney disease (ESKD) the kidneys no longer function appropriately. A technique needs to be found to mimic the way they work or they need to be replaced by means of transplantation. For many patients the choice of transplantation is seen as the ideal treatment for ESKD. However, this is not always possible because of the limited number of either cadaver or living donors available to provide kidneys to the population that needs to replacement. Many patients must therefore rely on replacement therapy. The bulk of this involves some form of dialysis therapy. There are a range of different types of dialysis including haemodialysis and peritoneal dialysis. These treatments are delivered in either a hospital or treatment centre or in some cases at home. The regimen of dialysis treatment is extremely onerous. It places great pressure on patients to attend treatments usually a number of times a week. In addition they have to adopt a specific diet to reduce the pressure on their kidneys. Most people who have ESKD commonly have an additional chronic condition. Conditions such as diabetes and high blood pressure often cause people to go into ESKD. This means that many patients with ESKD also have to follow the requirements and regimens of other conditions that are in their own way demanding.

This eBook focuses on the impact of this complex and exacting condition on patients and those that care for them. It also examines the economic impact of end - stage kidney disease and the healthcare policy implications of this disease. It provides comprehensive and thoughtful insights into the issues patients with ESKD confront. It is written by researchers with a well-rounded understanding of the characteristics and impact of ESKD. I can think of no better group to examine the consequences of ESKD on patients than the expert contributors to this eBook. For anyone involved in the treatment and management of end - stage kidney disease - professionals, patients and their families - this eBook provides essential reading.

Stanton Newman
City University London
United Kingdom

Foreword by Robert A. Cummins

Throughout the various stages of life, increasing levels of scientific and ethical attention are being directed to the consequences of medical intervention. The measures being studied are additional to the traditional indices of biological functioning and survival. Such monitoring is becoming especially important towards the end of life, where the cost of treatment ever rises in response to increasing technical sophistication. The downside to increasing longevity through such means is the burden of such treatments. What, then, is the balance between the duration of life gained and life quality? These critical contemporary questions are addressed in this compelling collection of chapters relating to End Stage Kidney Disease (ESKD), from diverse viewpoints.

Patients suffering from ESKD have to cope with many forms of adversity. Most obviously, their treatment is expensive so they bear an economic burden. The treatment is also inherently unpleasant, so they must bear the burden of pain and discomfort. Such constant feelings of malaise have knock-on consequences, such as a loss of motivation to engage in normal positive behaviors. This loss, in turn, is likely to exacerbate the severity of their condition through, for example, the loss of motivation to eat a good diet or to meet the requirements of demanding treatment regimens. But overshadowing all of these is the social cost of their condition. The disruption of normal social relationships with partner, family and friends can mean a devastating reduction in this major personal resource against adversity.

Understanding and ameliorating such negative outcomes is important for at least two reasons. One is a humanitarian concern with life quality. The other is the fact that loss of positive feelings leads to depression, which then works against the potential benefits afforded by the medical treatment. People who are despondent respond less positively to medical interventions. Moreover, without due care, their psychological condition also causes them to interact negatively with the world around them, causing an emotional downwards spiral as they lose social support and positive self-regard.

Measuring and interpreting such outcomes requires good instruments and theoretical understanding of the underlying psychological constructs. Two disciplines are intimately involved. Within medicine, such measurements are viewed within the context of health related quality of life, and many instruments have been created. Such measures constitute standardized self-reports of each patient's symptoms, both in terms of their medical condition and psychopathology. From within psychology, established scales have been created to measure levels of depression and stress, while more recent instruments measure levels of positive wellbeing.

All such measurements contribute important information for those who must make tough decisions. Does the life quality of the patient warrant continuation of the treatment, all things considered? Such decisions are made every day in money-stretched hospitals and will become more frequent as the economic reality of extending life becomes increasingly relevant. This fine collection of chapters adds important understanding to this crucial area of human intervention.

Robert A. Cummins

School of Psychology
Deakin University
Melbourne
Australia

PREFACE

Modern societies include increasing proportions of elderly people, with a resulting increase in the incidence and duration of chronic illnesses. Similarly, advanced age is considered a significant determinant of depression and poor quality of life. Additionally, the provision of therapies relevant to chronic diseases addresses the issues beyond the concept of cure, bringing to the center the need for a dignified quality of life of patients. An increased interest in quality of life is observed in patients who suffer from chronic diseases, including those with end-stage kidney disease. End-stage kidney disease patients have a high burden of disease affecting their quality of life and dramatically shortening their life expectancy. Therefore, exploring quality of life becomes an essential task in the management of this population. This volume provides a penetrating practical discussion to date of alternative approaches for comprehensively measuring the burden of end-stage kidney disease.

DISCLOSURE

The part of text has been taken from the article *J Clin Med Res.* **2011 3(3): 132–138**. (http://www.ncbi.nlm.nih.gov/pmc/articles/PMC3138410/)

Paraskevi Theofilou
Sotiria Hospital for Thoracic Diseases
Athens
Greece

&

Center for Research and Technology
Department of Kinesiology
Health & Quality of Life Research Group
Trikala
Thessaly
Greece

List of Contributors

Alden Y. Lai

Graduate School of Medicine, School of Public Health, University of Tokyo, Tokyo, Japan

Anne Vereerstraeten

CHU André Vésale, Montigny-Le-Tilleul, Chimay, Tunisia

Anne-Marie Bogaert

AZ Sint Elisabeth, Zottegem, Belgium

Athena Kalokairinou

University of Athens, Nursing Department, Athens, Greece

Barbara Barcaccia

Associazione di Psicologia Cognitiva, Rome, Italy

Christina Karatzaferi

Department of Kinesiology, Center for Research and Technology, Thessaly, Greece; Department of Physical Education and Sport Science, University of Thessaly, Greece

Constantinos M. Togas

Ministry of Justice, Hellas, Greece

Cynthia Russell

University of Missouri-Kansas City, School of Nursing, USA

Georgios K. Tzitzikos

General Hospital of Corinth, Renal Department, Hellas, Greece

Giorgos K. Sakkas

Department of Kinesiology, Center for Research and Technology, Thessaly, Greece; Department of Physical Education and Sport Science, University of Thessaly, Greece

Guy Van Roost

St. Jan Hospital Brussels, Belgium

Haikel A. Lim

Department of Psychology, National University of Singapore, Singapore

Helen Panagiotaki

"A. Fleming" General Hospital of Melissia, Melissia, Athens, Greece

Josipa Radic

Department of Internal Medicine, University Hospital Center Split, University of Split School of Medicine, Split, Croatia

Karin Caekelbergh

Health Economics and Outcomes Research, IMS Health, Brussels, Belgium

Katarina Dodig Curkovic

Department of Psychiatry, University Hospital Center Osijek, University of Osijek School of Medicine, Osijek, Croatia

Koen Bouman

ZNA, Middelheim, Antwerp, Belgium

Konstadina Griva

Faculty of Arts & Social Sciences, Department of Psychology, National University of Singapore, Singapore

Maria Athanasopoulou

University of Athens, Nursing Department, Athens, Greece

Maria Malliarou

University of Athens, Nursing Department, Athens, Greece

Mario Schurgers

AZ St. Jan, Brugge, Belgium

Mark Lamotte

Health Economics and Outcomes Research, IMS Health, Brussels, Belgium

Max Dratwa

CHU Brugmann, Brussels, Belgium

Michelle L. Matteson

University of Missouri, Department of Gastroenterology and Hepatology, USA

Mislav Radic

Department of Internal Medicine, University Hospital Center Split, University of Split School of Medicine, Split, Croatia

Pantelis Sarafidis

1st Medical Department, Aristotle University, Thessaloniki, Greece

Paraskevi Theofilou

Sotiria Hospital for Thoracic Diseases, Athens, Greece; Center for Research and Technology, Department of Kinesiology, Health & Quality of Life Research Group, Trikala, Thessaly, Greece; Sotiria Hospital for Thoracic Diseases, Athens, Greece

Pavlos Malindretos

Department of Nephrology, Peritoneal Dialysis Section, Achillopouleion General Hospital, Volos, Greece

Pierre Dupont

CHU Tivoli, La Louvière, Belgium

Remi Hombrouckx

AZ Zusters van Barmhartigheid, Ronse, Belgium

Sofia Zyga

University of Peloponnese, Nursing Department, Sparta, Greece

Stamatina Zili

Department of Internal Medicine, Papageorgiou General Hospital, Thessaloniki, Greece

Stefania S. Grigoriou

Department of Kinesiology, Center for Research and Technology and Department of Physical Education and Sport Science, University of Thessaly, Greece

Suzanne Laplante

EMEA Health Outcomes chez Baxter Healthcare, Baxter World Trade SA/NV, Belgium

Xavier Warling

Center Hospital Régionale Citadelle, Liège, Belgium

2

CHAPTER 1

Introduction to Outcomes Assessment in End - Stage Kidney Disease

Paraskevi Theofilou[1,2,*]

[1]Sotiria Hospital for Thoracic Diseases, Athens, Greece and [2]Center for Research and Technology, Department of Kinesiology, Health & Quality of Life Research Group, Trikala, Thessaly, Greece

Abstract: End - stage kidney disease (ESKD) is characterized by deterioration of renal function, which ends fatally in uremia, and this is detected by multisystem manifestations. The present book evaluates the state of the science in end - stage kidney disease outcomes assessment and offers perspectives on what is required to advance the field. The chapters collectively cover a diverse set of topics, which are examined in a sequence suggested by the broad section heading below. Developed as stand - alone documents, the chapters can be read in any order. Each chapter presents a number of findings and the previews below provide only a favor of the full range of results.

Keywords: End - stage kidney disease, ESKD, outcomes, chapter, findings, section, preview, topics.

OUTCOMES ASSESSMENT IN ESKD

Chronic kidney disease (CKD), also known as chronic renal disease, is a progressive loss in renal function over a period of months or years. The symptoms of worsening kidney function are non - specific, and might include feeling generally unwell and experiencing a reduced appetite. Often, CKD is diagnosed as a result of screening of people known to be at risk of kidney problems, such as those with high blood pressure or diabetes and those with a blood relative with CKD. Chronic kidney disease may also be identified when it leads to one of its recognized complications, such as cardiovascular disease, anemia or pericarditis (National Kidney Foundation, 2002). Recent professional guidelines classify the severity of chronic kidney disease in five stages, with stage 1 being the mildest and usually causing few symptoms and stage 5 being a severe illness with poor

Address correspondence to Paraskevi Theofilou: Sotiria Hospital for Thoracic Diseases, Athens, Greece; Center for Research and Technology, Department of Kinesiology, Health & Quality of Life Research Group, Trikala, Thessaly, Greece; Tel: +0030 6977441502, Fax: +0030 2106221435; E-mail: theofi@otenet.gr; paraskevi.theofilou@gmail.com

life expectancy if untreated. Stage 5 CKD is often called End - Stage Kidney Disease (ESKD) and is synonymous with the now outdated terms chronic kidney failure (CKF) or chronic renal failure (CRF) (National Kidney Foundation, 2002).

ESKD is characterized by deterioration of renal function, which ends fatally in uremia, and this is detected by multisystem manifestations (Nettina, 2001). Schena *et al.,* (2001) indicated that the clinical signs and symptoms of ESKD are highly variable because of inter - individual differences and co-morbidity (hypertension and diabetes mellitus). The first abnormalities indicated by the patient are nocturia and polyuria along with loss of performance. This is accompanied by hypertension and its sequelae (headache, dyspnea, left heart failure, coronary heart disease) and by edema. The terminal stage is characterized by hiccups, muscular twitching, lethargy, somnolence, and coma.

ESKD can be treated by extracorporeal blood purification, peritoneal dialysis (PD), or transplantation. It is important to recognize that different therapies are not competing and need to be utilized in an integrated manner, together with transplantation, to enhance patient outcome. The proportion of patients on PD or haemodialysis (HD) varies considerably from country to country. The choice appears to be more related to nonmedical factors such as finance, reimbursement, physician biases, and social mores (Nissenson *et al.*, 1997).

Patients suffering from ESKD have to cope with many adversities, *e.g.*, physical symptoms, limitations in food and fluid intake, changes in their body image, work and economic status, social roles, activity levels, self-image, health status, and normal routines, while their control over treatment cannot always be predicted (Theofilou, 2012; Theofilou, 2012a; Theofilou, 2013; Theofilou, Synodinou & Panagiotaki, 2013a). Such constraints are expected to affect the patients' lives and their physical and social functioning, leading them to reconsider their personal and professional goals within the context of living with a chronic illness (Ginieri - Coccossis *et al.*, 2008; Theofilou, 2012b; Theofilou, 2012c).

Psychological, as well as social adaptation during the early periods of the progression of renal disease is particularly essential for ESKD patients and the family. Depression and anxiety about the unknown, the prospect of starting replacement therapy, sexual dysfunction, and loss of income, vocation, and social role may all be important in the development of maladjustment (Geenberg *et al.*, 1998). Psychological status of ESKD patients must be monitored to prevent psychological problems. The mode of replacement therapy is chosen according to the patient personality and life situation. Counseling would enhance patient compliance while psychotherapy and drug therapy is initiated in case of psychological problems such as depression, anxiety or dementia (Daugirdas *et al.*, 2001). On the other hand, ESKD patients must be assessed by social worker in order to detect social problems developing as a result of the disease, and enhance social support and social interaction through family education and counseling.

This book is intended to host the new and existing findings on Outcomes Assessment in end-stage kidney disease as well as to present the most recent developments and ideas in the field with regards to the individual patient care. "Outcomes research" may be defined generally as the scientific field devoted to measuring and interpreting the impact of medical conditions and health care on individuals as well as populations. In the area of end-stage kidney disease, "outcomes research" describes, interprets and predicts the impact of various influences, especially (but not exclusively) interventions on "final" endpoints. Such final endpoints may include health-related quality of life, as captured through either generic (non-disease specific), general end-stage kidney disease, or end-stage kidney disease site-specific measures, health locus of control, level of adherence and economic burden, through cost analysis or cost-effectiveness studies, as felt by patients, caregivers, payers or society at large.

Organization of the eBook

The present eBook evaluates the state of the science in end - stage kidney disease outcomes assessment and offers perspectives on what is required to advance the field. The chapters collectively cover a diverse set of topics, which are examined in a sequence suggested by the broad section heading below. Developed as stand - alone documents, the chapters can be read in any order. Each chapter presents a number of findings and the previews below provide only a favor of the full range of results.

Health - Related Quality of Life in End - Stage Kidney Disease: Concept and Measurement

Barbara Barcaccia discusses alternative definitions and domains for health - related quality of life, emphasizing the distinction between quality of life (QoL) and health - related quality of life (HRQoL). She poses some very crucial questions with regards to this definition like *"Which are the conditions that make life good?"* or *"Is it possible to decide the criteria which make a life valuable or worthwhile living?"* But defining what HRQoL is involves also ethical considerations: when decisions about severely ill or disabled patients need to be taken, having a clear idea of what a good/bad quality of life is becomes essential.

Stefania Grigoriou, Christina Karatzaferi and Giorgos Sakkas analyze the use of the most common generic and specific (kidney disease) HRQoL measures in chronic kidney disease (CKD) outcomes research. The chapter reviews the development and psychometric properties of these measures. It also discusses the criteria that any QoL instrument should meet in order to be functional in the clinical practice. Finally, various interventions are discussed, such as the influence of exercise and cognitive behaviour therapy on the psychosocial status of CKD patients.

Assessing Health - Related Quality of Life in Patients Undergoing Dialysis

Haikel A. Lim and Konstadina Griva address thoroughly QoL issues in end - stage kidney disease (ESKD). They first investigate the various issues surrounding QoL in dialysis research. Then, they review the empirical findings and limitations in this area. They end by proposing applications of QoL research in clinical settings, and examine empirical research that might potentially assist patients with decision-making for different treatment modalities.

Health - Related Quality of Life Issues Among Kidney Transplanted Patients

Pavlos Malindretos, Stamatina. Zili and Pantelis Sarafidis discuss thoroughly HRQoL issues in kidney transplanted patients. Specifically, a narrative review lies which aims to present to the reader as many different approaches as possible regarding correlation between kidney transplantation and HRQoL. An additional effort was made so that QoL of children and adults, living relative and non - relative donors, men and women would be incorporated in their chapter.

Josipa Radic, Mislav Radic and Katarina Dodig Curkovic examine the cognitive function in end - stage kidney disease (ESKD) patients. Specifically, they investigate the prevalence of cognitive impairment in these patients as well as the factors which may contribute to their cognitive impairment. They also examine the relation of various clinical variables, like dialysis dose, hemodialysis process and dialysis modality, to the cognitive function. They conclude that cognitive impairment in ESKD patients prior and post-transplantation is important area of health and that periodic assessment of an ESKD patient's cognitive function should be one of the basic parameters to be considered on evaluating outcomes after kidney transplantation.

Dialysis Patients' Adherence to Treatment and Interventions to Improve it

Alden Y. Lai and Konstadina Griva focused on the topic of treatment adherence in patients undergoing dialysis, outlining recent conceptualisation approached, relevant measures and criteria, and summarising literature on adherence rates, further offering a brief overview of related interventions. They have also outlined the broad categories of demographic, clinical and psychosocial factors affecting treatment adherence.

Michelle L. Matteson and Cynthia Russell have systematically reviewed intervention studies targeting treatment, diet, fluid, and medication adherence in adult hemodialysis patients from 2007 to May 2012. The Cumulative Index of Nursing and Allied Health Literature (CINAHL), MEDLINE, PsychINFO, and all Evidence-Based Medicine (EBM) Reviews (Cochran DSR, ACP Journal Club, DARE, and CCTR) were searched to identify studies testing efficacy of interventions to improve adherence to treatment, fluid, medication and diet adherence in adult hemodialysis patients. In summary, eleven studies (two randomized controlled trial and nine quasi-experimental studies) were identified attempting to enhance hemodialysis adherence.

Measuring the Experience and Needs of End - Stage Kidney Disease Patients' Caregivers

Georgios K. Tzitzikos and Constantinos M. Togas have drawn on the key literature in this field as identified by psychiatric, medical and social sciences databases, with the aim to conduct a systematic review which explores the psychological burden and QoL in ESKD adults and children patients' caregivers. The authors describe very thoroughly the studies' findings indicating the experience and needs of these people.

Sofia Zyga, Maria Malliarou, Maria Athanasopoulou and Athena Kalokairinou have addressed another crucial part related to the ESKD patients' caregivers. They discuss the relationship between loss and grief that renal nurses experience and stress management. Work in dialysis units involves intensive and long-term contact with patients who are often frustrated or depressive, as well as confrontation with suffering and death, staff cuts and dealing with ever developing highly modern technologies.

Assessing the Economic Burden of End - Stage Kidney Disease

The need to reduce cost in combination with the existence of options in every act or function that requires financial sacrifices makes economic evaluation as a necessary methodological tool, which helps specialists to make rational decisions. Paraskevi Theofilou and Helen Panagiotaki aimed to evaluate the dialysis cost at a private clinic in 2007 in Athens. Specifically, a comparative cost analysis between bicarbonate dialysis and haemodiafiltration is performed. The present work through the economic evaluation for one of the two methods of dialysis, aspires to contribute to or at least to pique interest in developing further reflection and study of an alternative form of financing. Moreover, the calculation of the cost of treatment can be the starting point to perform cost-effectiveness studies, enabling benchmarking the effectiveness and efficiency of these.

Max Dratwa, Anne-Marie Bogaert, Koen Bouman, Xavier Warling, Remi Hombrouckx, Mario Schurgers, Pierre Dupont, Anne Vereerstraeten, Guy Van Roost, Karin Caekelbergh, Mark Lamotte and Suzanne Laplante assess the economic burden of patients requiring dialysis to the Belgian public healthcare payer (*e.g.*, dialysis procedure; hospitalizations; ambulatory care; medications; transport). This study provides further evidence that home modalities, such as peritoneal dialysis, could help reduce the economic burden of dialysis on the healthcare budget.

Research and Policy Implications

The focus of this section is on outcomes data development. Paraskevi Theofilou has addressed the importance of the use of patient reported outcomes (PRO) measures by the pharmaceutical industry. Does the industry, however, make full use of its PRO data? Companies to consider all potential means of making interested parties aware of relevant information are required for a PRO strategy for a new compound. She concludes that in order to keep pace with developments in emerging methods of communication, strategies for dissemination of key messages will need to evolve.

CONCLUSIONS

Understanding how a disease and its associated health care interventions affect the lives of individuals is important whatever the medical condition, but especially so for the diseases that are chronic or incurable and for which treatments often have long - lasting consequences. For this reason, end-stage kidney disease provides an exceptionally compelling model for examining the impact of disease on individual well-being. Along with survival and other types of clinical outcome, the functioning and well - being that characterize end - stage kidney disease patients are important indicators of the effectiveness of the medical care that they receive. Chronic dialysis, peritoneal dialysis and kidney transplantation are miracles of medical technology, and the ability of these technologies to sustain lives is of unquestioned significance. However, medical effectiveness is increasingly viewed from multiple prospectives that include more than patients survival rates and clinical outcome. Patients' functional status, quality of life and satisfaction along with treatment costs also determine the effectiveness of care. All these factors need to be clearly understood by the hospital staff to enable them to support the patient in an individualized way.

The readers of this eBook mainly include health professionals who are engaged with the care of end-stage kidney disease patients *e.g.,* physicians, nurses, psychologists *etc.* as well as students in the fields of medicine, nursing, psychology or social work. The contents can be also useful for health economists and health policy makers. It is essential to remember that health - related quality of life is a very important tool for the evaluation of health policies.

My hope is that readers will have a sense of where the field is now and will be encouraged to participate in its future growth.

ACKNOWLEDGEMENTS

None Declared.

CONFLICT OF INTEREST

None Declared.

REFERENCES

Daugirdas, J. T., Blake, P. G., & Ing, T. S. (2001). Handbook of dialysis. (3rd ed.) Philadelphia: USA: Lippincott Williams & Wilkins.

Ginieri-Coccossis M, Theofilou P, Synodinou C, Tomaras V, Soldatos C. (2008). Quality of life, mental health and health beliefs in haemodialysis and peritoneal dialysis patients: Investigating differences in early and later years of treatment. BioMed Central Nephrology, 9, 1-26.

Greenberg, A., Cheung, A. K., Coffmann, T. M., Falk, R. J., & Jennette, J. C. (1998). Primer on kidney diseases. (2nd ed.) San Diego: California: Academic Press.

National Kidney Foundation (2002). K/DOQI clinical practice guidelines for chronic kidney disease. http://www.kidney.org/professionals/KDOQI/guidelines_ckd. Retrieved 2008-06-29.

Nettina, S. M. (2001). The lippincott manual of nursing practice. (7th ed.) Philadelphia: USA: Lippincott Williams & Wilkins.

Nissenson AR, Prichard SS, Cheng IK, Gokal R, Kubota M, Maiorca R, Riella MC, Rottembourg J, Stewart JH. (1997). ESRD modality selection into the 21st century: the importance of nonmedical factors. ASAIO J 43(3): 143-150.

Schena, F. P., Davison, A. M., Koomans, H. A., Grunfeld, J.-P., Valderrabano, F., Van der Woude, F. J. *et al.,* (2001). Nephrology. Maidenhead, Berkshire: England: McGraw-Hill International (UK) Ltd.

Theofilou P. (2012). Self - reported functional status: an important predictor of mental health outcomes among chronic dialysis patients. European Journal of Psychological Assessment, DOI 10.1027/1015-5759/a000155.

Theofilou P. (2012a). The effect of sociodemographic features and beliefs about medicines on adherence to chronic kidney disease treatment, Journal of Clinical Research & Bioethics, 3(2), 1-5.

Theofilou P. (2012b). Medication adherence in Greek hemodialysis patients: The contribution of depression and health cognitions. International Journal of Behavioral Medicine, on line first published, DOI 10.1007/s12529-012-9231-8.

Theofilou P. (2012c). Quality of life and mental health in hemodialysis and peritoneal dialysis patients: the role of health beliefs. International Urology and Nephrology, 44(1), 245-253.

Theofilou P. (2013). Association of insomnia with kidney disease quality of life reported by patients on maintenance dialysis, Psychology, Health & Medicine, 18(1), 70-78.

Theofilou, P., Synodinou, C., Panagiotaki H. (2013a). Undergoing Haemodialysis - A qualitative study to investigate the lived experiences of patients. Europe's Journal of Psychology, 9, 19-32.

CHAPTER 2

Definitions and Domains of Health - Related Quality of Life

Barbara Barcaccia[*]

Associazione di Psicologia Cognitiva, Rome, Italy

Abstract: Healthcare in the 21st century has moved from a disease-centred perspective to a patient-centred one, in which the concept of quality of life plays a crucial role. Nowadays, with an ageing population throughout most of the world and an increased life expectancy, there is a large number of individuals living with physical and/or mental chronic illnesses/disabilities. Therefore, the focus of medicine has shifted towards the quality of survival, and not only on the mere length of life. For these reasons health - related quality of life (HRQoL) has become an important field of study in medical care. The present work focuses on the definitions and domains regarding HRQoL. But defining what quality of life is involves also ethical considerations: when decisions about severely ill or disabled patients need to be taken, having a clear idea of what a good/bad quality of life is becomes essential. Clinicians and researchers in the health care should be aware of the importance of HRQoL and its implications. Indeed the concept of HRQoL allows professional caregivers to understand the patient's evaluations and perceptions of his/her illness/disability and of the related treatments. Moreover it allows comparisons among different interventions and their respective effectiveness.

Keywords: Health-related quality of life, domains, definitions, models, acceptance, ethical issues.

DEFINITION AND DOMAINS OF HRQoL

What is "quality of life"? A clear and shared definition of this construct is very hard to find. This difficulty depends also, but not only, on the fact that QoL research has been conducted on an ample range of subjects: indeed it is a concept which has overspread almost all fields of knowledge and life. This term is amply used in everyday life, from commercials to politics, as well as in the context of research in a great many disciplines, from psychology to economics (Farquhar, 1995).

*Address correspondence to Barbara Barcaccia: Psy.D. Associazione di Psicologia Cognitiva, Rome, Italy; Tel: +39 0644704193; Fax: +39 0644360720; E -mail: barbara.barcaccia@uniroma1.it

In a way "It is also a vague concept; it is multidimensional and theoretically incorporates all aspects of an individual's life" (Bowling, 2001, p. 2).

As highlighted by Bowling (1995) the expression "quality of life" can refer to a series of different meanings that are as diverse as good physical health, life satisfaction and happiness. QoL can be considered the degree of satisfaction of, *e.g.*, psychological, physical, social needs, such as safety, belongingness, freedom, comfort, *etc.*

In a more subjective (phenomenological) perspective, it can be seen as the way an individual evaluates one's life: *"consistent with this view, evaluations of quality of life must evolve from the viewer, the person whose life's quality about which we are concerned"* (Ziller, 1974, p. 303). From this standpoint, despite the possibility of assessing the different positive and negative life events and conditions of the individual, it is mainly the personal experiencing of these events and the meaning attached to them that explains what quality of life is (Ziller, 1974). In psychology this perspective is embraced by the cognitivist approach, according to which wellbeing depends on the individual's interpretation and appraisal of external and internal events (Beck, 1976; Ellis, 1994; Barcaccia, 2008; Saliani, Barcaccia & Mancini, 2011).

Defining what quality of life is can be considered also an ethical issue: when decisions about severely ill or disabled patients have to be taken, having a clear idea of what a good/bad health-related quality of life is becomes essential.

As rightly pointed out by Chen, Li, & Kochen (2005) the consequence of advances in medicine is a growing number of individuals living with chronic diseases and disabilities. This means there is a need to modify the paradigm regarding how we evaluate outcomes of illness and care: *"Is it worthwhile to keep a comatose person alive on a respirator? Is renal transplant a better treatment than haemodialysis for patients with renal failure? Is one particular health care delivery system better for patients with chronic diseases than another? Traditional indicators like mortality rates and objective clinical parameters are no longer adequate for answering these questions"* (Chen *et al.*, 2005, p. 936). Quality of life is, therefore, a crucial concept "when it is necessary to decide about a person's life, that is, in the context of withholding or withdrawal of life-sustaining medical intervention" (Marcos Del Cano, 2001, p. 91).

And as a consequence appropriate instruments of evaluations should be available. Reliable HRQoL instruments are extremely important in chronic conditions where a major objective of management is to arrest or reverse the decline in function and quality of life. (Gurková, 2011, p. 191).

Moreover, as noted by Lin, Lin & Fan (2012), there are at least three reasons why scholars and clinicians should pay attention to the concept of HRQoL. Firstly, it is an important way to understand the patient's perspective on his/her illness or disability and the applied treatment. Secondly it helps to understand how the normal process of adjustment to disease develops and how treatment works, and conversely, to detect when the process is stuck, when it becomes abnormal and when a modification in the treatment is necessary. Thirdly, HRQoL allows sound and reliable comparisons among different interventions and their respective effectiveness.

QUALITY OF LIFE *VS.* HEALTH-RELATED QUALITY OF LIFE

As noted by Lin *et al.,* (2012), although QoL and HRQoL are often used as synonymous, the two definitions refer to different concepts: QoL is a broad concept covering all aspects of human life, whereas HRQoL focuses on the effects of illness and specifically on the impact of treatment on QoL (Lin *et al.*, 2012, p. 1).

QoL is a broader concept, when compared to HRQoL, since it includes the evaluation of non health-related features of life, while HRQoL has been defined as quality of life connected to the individual's health or disease status. In particular, which is the impact of illness and of the treatment on the quality of life? The concept of HRQoL helps to understand the distinction between the aspects of life related to health and those that are beyond the compass of health care, such as education, social and geographical environment, *etc.* (Theofilou, 2012).

HRQoL differentiates the aspects of life directly related to health from those that are not comprised within the compass of health care (Ferrans, 2005).

QoL can be seen in terms of the gap between an ideal life and the actual one: *"Quality of life therefore, measures the difference, at a particular moment in time, between the hopes and expectations of the individual and that individual's present experiences"* (Calman, 1984, p. 125).

Malkina-Pykh and Pykh (2008) consider QoL as a measure of how positively or negatively individuals perceive their lives. In the Authors' perspective QoL is a measure of well-being, affected by three main domains, built environment QoL, social environment QoL and economic environment QoL. The built QoL is where one lives: house, surroundings, available facilities, and infrastructure. The social environment QoL involves friends, family, entertainment, health and education level. The economic environment QoL regards money, how money is spent, employment/unemployment.

According to Calman (1984) *"QoL depends on present lifestyle, past experience, hopes for the future, dreams and ambitions. Quality of life must include all areas of life and experience and take into account the impact of illness and treatment. A good quality of life can be said to be present when the hopes of an individual are matched and fulfilled by experience. The opposite is also true: a poor quality of life occurs when the hopes do not meet with the experience"* (Calman, 1984, p. 124-125).

As above shown, there are some interpretations of the QoL construct that include every aspect of life, from employment to religion, but within the health care field not all the human concerns can be encompassed (Lin *et al.*, 2012). This is the reason why this construct in health care is more easily described as health-related quality of life, even though it has been maintained that "the concept of health related quality of life is an equally nebulous concept" (Bowling, 1995, p. 1448), as QoL sometimes appears to be.

HRQoL has been also distinguished from health status: even though the latter can influence HRQoL, it cannot be considered the same domain, because health status *"assesses physical and mental symptoms, disability, and social dysfunction related to a health situation in a mere descriptive way, lacking judgments about their impact on the individual's well being and expectations"* (Martinez-Martin &

Kurtis, 2012, p. 105). Also Lin *et al.*, (2012) highlight the distinction between health status and HRQoL.

HRQoL can be considered as the patient's subjective perception of the impact of his/her disease and its treatment on the daily life, psychological, physical and social functioning.

DEFINITIONS OF HEALTH - RELATED QUALITY OF LIFE

As noted by Gurková (2011), there is a general consensus in the conceptualisation of HRQoL as a multidimensional construct, composed of physical, psychological and social features of health. These domains attempt to cover the challenging and far-reaching WHO definition of health: *"A state of complete physical, mental and social well-being and not merely the absence of disease or infirmity"* (WHO Group, 1995, p. 1403).

In this perspective it is important to acknowledge that HRQoL does not depend only upon physical health. In fact there might be individuals with poor physical health that evaluate their HRQoL as good. "*Most health professionals recognize that diagnostic measures, such as ejection fractions and viral loads, correlate poorly with how well the patients functions at a "macro" level, from walking and stretching to getting and holding a job, let alone with how satisfied the patient is with his health or his life*" (Wasserman, Bickenbach & Wachbroit, 2005, p. 6).

HRQoL has been described as "the extent to which one's usual or expected physical, emotional and social well-being are affected by a medical condition or its treatment" (Cella, 1996, p. 234). Testa and Simonson (1996) define HRQOL as the "physical, psychological and social domains of health, seen as distinct areas that are influenced by a person's experiences, beliefs, expectations and perceptions" (p. 835). Benito-León *et al.*, (2011) consider that "*HRQoL is a concept that involves those aspects of quality of life or function, which is influenced by health status and is based on dimensions (i.e., physical, psychological, and social aspects), which can be measured*" (Benito- León *et al.*, 2011, p. 676).

In the following part I shall follow Gurková's summary (2011):

HRQoL is multidimensional, in the sense that each individual can refer to different characteristics of his/her life when reflecting upon their own HRQoL. This happens because the features of this construct are varied and include physical, emotional, psychological, social and spiritual aspects of life.

HRQoL is dynamic, in the sense that it will vary over time. Let's consider how an individual's priorities, goals and expectations can change over different phases of life. Emotional stability, *e.g.*, could be considered an important achievement in adulthood, but not in adolescence, or vice-versa.

HRQoL is subjective and value-based: each individual rates his/her own quality of life from a perspective that can only be subjective, *i.e.,* based on one's feelings, expectations, desires and values (Pallini, Bove & Laghi, 2011).

Every human being uses a personal standard to evaluate a status as desirable or undesirable. Personal evaluation of one's HRQoL is absolutely necessary if a professional caregiver wants to really understand which the impact is of, *e.g.*, a chronic illness on a person's life: in truth this kind of evaluation is something very different from the "objective" evaluation of a patient's health status.

According to Bowling (2001) there's been in the last decades a growing tendency in the field of experiential social indicators to focus on the importance of the subjective wellbeing. The outcomes of this research have shown that objective variables, as opposed to subjective ones, *"account for relatively little of the variance in happiness, life satisfaction and well-being, thus leading to more emphasis on the importance of subjective feelings of independence, control and autonomy as predictors of well-being"* (Bowling, 2001, p. 2). In other words, ten people affected by the same illness, no matter how severe, might have ten different qualities of life. But literature also shows, *e.g.*, that also family members (partners, caregivers) of severely ill patients can be highly distressed because of their dear one' diagnosis (Segrin, Badger, Dorros, Meek & Lopez, 2007), and in some cases their QoL is worse than that of patients (Barcaccia, Mismetti & Saliani, 2010; Mismetti & Barcaccia, 2011).

"What HRQoL measurements hope to capture are patients' subjective perceptions and assessments of their health. These perceptions and assessments cannot be

measured by blood testing, electroencephalography, MRI, or any other "objective" testing" (Wilson, 2004, p. 434).

HRQoL involves the individual's perceptions of both positive and negative dimensions. If we consider that the ultimate goal for a clinician that wants to assess another individual's quality of life is to promote his/her wellbeing, it is clear that the evaluation cannot comprise only the negative features such as deficits, loss of abilities, psychopathology, functional limitations, but should also include positive aspects, such as the overcoming of challenges posed by chronic disease, becoming role-models for others, a renewed commitment to spiritual values, *etc.*

"HRQoL is a double-sided concept that includes both positive and negative aspects of health. The negative aspect includes disease and dysfunctions, whereas the positive aspect encompasses feelings of mental and physical wellbeing, full functioning, physical fitness, adjustment, and efficiency of the mind and body" (Lin *et al.*, 2012, p. 1)

When an individual reports, *e.g.*, low back pain, professional caregivers are supposed to assess the severity of the presented problem, potential comorbidity with other syndromes/symptoms, in addition to what kinds of activities prevents the person from doing, which types of movements are hindered, how the social functioning is affected by the low back pain, how he/she is coping with the pain and how these problems influence the individual's sense of wellbeing (Wilson, 2004).

DOMAINS OF HEALTH - RELATED QUALITY OF LIFE

HRQoL is generally considered as subjective, dynamic, and multidimensional. The dimensions included are mainly physical, psychological, social, and spiritual factors (Bakas *et al.*, 2012).

Berzon, Hays, & Shumaker (1993) identified the following dimensions of HRQOL: physical functioning, psychological, functioning, social functioning, role activities, overall life satisfaction, and perceptions of health status.

According to Chen *et al.*, (2005), "function" is the most important dimension of HRQoL. It should comprise physical, social and role function. But there also other significant domains, such as mental health and general health perception. Vitality, pain and cognitive function are also important domains of HRQoL (Wilson & Cleary, 1995).

As pointed out by Guyatt *et al.*, (1993), HRQoL is a concept that tries to embrace the spirit of the WHO definition of health (WHO, 1948) by including both personal health status and social wellbeing when assessing health: "... *individuals' perception of their position in life in the context of the culture and value system in which they live and in relation to their goals, expectations and standards and concerns. It is a broad ranging concept affected in a complex way by the person's physical health, psychological state, level of independence, social relationships, and their relationship to salient features of their environment.*" (definition of "quality of life" according to the WHO Group, 1995, p. 1403).

Evaluation of HRQoL should be subjective, that is the person being assessed rates his own status (Lam, 1997).

It has been rightly stated that WHO's definition of health (WHO Group, 1995) allows a more holistic view of HRQoL, resulting particularly important when applied to individuals with disabilities: it is not just a matter of the presence/absence of disability, but other factors have to be taken into account. *Presence of disability is not automatically equated with decreased health-related quality of life. Just as two people with the same disability are as different as any two people, so too is the health-related impact that disability imposes on quality of life.* (Sheppard-Jones, 2003, p. 4). Actually, an illness might influence one's life in many different ways. The most intuitive one is the negative impact on mood, functioning, *etc.* But, even though it might sound strange, in some cases the quality of life might be even enhanced and the so-called benefits of illness could occur (Calman, 1984).

In an interesting study Bowling (1995) wanted to find the population norms on the life's domains that people perceived to be important, in relation to QoL and HRQoL. The purpose was to investigate people's positive and negative domains, by simply asking individuals about what was important in their lives. QoL was operationalized as the things people consider as important in their lives, either good or bad. Respondents could state as many things as they wished, and afterwards up to five of them were coded. Participants were also asked to rank the mentioned items in hierarchical order, from the most important to the less important, and to assess their current status for each of them against a categorical scale. They were also asked to rate their overall life on a similar scale. The results showed that respondents were most likely to select as the first most important thing in their lives "relationships with family or relatives", followed by their "own health", the "health of another person" and "finances/standard of living/housing".

In a recent and challenging article on these issues, Bakas *et al.,* (2012) have conducted a thorough research on the most frequent HRQoL models used in the literature over the last years. In particular the Authors have focused on English language articles published between January 1, 1999 and August 31, 2010. The main purpose of their work was to identify which models are mostly used and to provide a critical analysis of those models. Results showed that the most common HRQoL models used in the scientific literature were those by Wilson and Cleary (1995), by the World Health Organization (WHO) and by Ferrans and colleagues (2005).

After a very detailed analysis of each model, the Authors (Bakas *et al.,* 2012) conclude that the revision of Wilson and Cleary's (1995) model by Ferrans, Zerwic, Wilbur, and Larson (2005) might be considered a very valid option, suitable for any health care discipline, because it provides clear and consistent conceptual and operational definitions, can explain well the relationships among variables, and constitutes a good guide for hypothesis generation. In this model the interaction among five different variables are illustrated: 1) Biological function (laboratory tests, physical examination, *etc.*) 2) Symptoms (physical and psychological symptoms, such as pain and depression) 3) Functional status (ability to perform certain tasks) 4) General health perceptions (individuals' subjective appraisal of their current health.) 5) Overall quality of life. The model takes also into account individual (*e.g.,* age, gender, *etc.*) and environmental characteristics (*e.g.,* social support).

Bakas *et al.,* (2012) also highlight that an explicit assumption of this model is that understanding relationships among the considered variables will lead to the development of optimally effective **clinical interventions**. They conclude that from their review emerge two main findings. Firstly, over the decade 1999-2010 there has been little consistency regarding HRQoL models within the literature: most of the reviewed articles used an already existing model as a guide, but many of them "mixed" different models, so that the terminology used to describe the same HRQoL concepts vastly varied. This makes cross-study comparisons very difficult to conduct. Secondly, it is important for researchers to choose one of the three (above-mentioned) most commonly used global models, because this would contribute to gather a coherent body of evidence, which is fundamental in order to enhance further HRQOL science. As already mentioned, the revision of the Wilson and Cleary's model by Ferrans, Zerwic, Wilbur, and Larson (2005) might be a very good choice according to Bakas *et al.*, (2012), because it provides clear and consistent conceptual and operational definitions, can explain well the relationships among variables, and constitutes a good guide for hypothesis generation. The Authors conclude their accurate review by stating the importance of using an already existing global model, so that it will be possible to compare HRQoL across studies and populations, contribute to the development of more intervention studies, and more quickly advance the science in the area of HRQOL (Bakas *et al.*, 2012).

CONCLUSIONS

Health-related quality of life is a fundamental concept in the field of health care. Important decisions regarding the lives of human beings are taken on the basis of these considerations: has this individual a good HRQoL? Which are the conditions that make life good? Is it possible to decide the criteria which make a life valuable or worthwhile living? The answers to these questions are ethically crucial, because they can determine either the withholding or the withdrawal of life-sustaining medical treatments.

Investigating a patient's HRQoL means reaching a better understanding of the patient's evaluations and reactions to his/her illness. As a matter of fact, we can consider HRQoL as the patient's subjective perception of the impact that the illness/disability and its treatments has on his/her life.

It is a multidimensional concept, which includes physical, emotional, psychological, spiritual and social aspects of life. It is a dynamic construct and it can vary over time, according to the individual's priorities, goals and expectations, which are likely to change over different phases of life. HRQoL is also subjective and value-based, because each human being evaluates quality of life from his/her own peculiar perspective, determined by one's feelings, expectations, beliefs, desires and values.

Literature has demonstrated so far that quality of life has not only to do with good physical health. Enormous ethical implications stem from these studies, and every professional caregiver in the healthcare system should give these issues serious consideration.

ACKNOWLEDGEMENTS

None Declared.

CONFLICT OF INTEREST

None Declared.

REFERENCES

Bakas T., McLennon S.M., Carpenter J.S., Buelow J.M., Otte J.L., Hanna K.M., Ellett M.L., Hadler K.A., Welch J.L. (2012). Systematic review of health-related quality of life models. Health and Quality of Life Outcomes, 10:134. Available from: http://www.hqlo.com/content/pdf/1477-7525-10-134.pdf [accessed 20th November 2012].

Barcaccia, B., Esposito, G., Matarese, M., Bertolaso, M., Elvira, M., De Marinis M.G. (2013). Defining quality of life: a wild-goose chase?, Europe's Journal of Psychology, special issue Quality of Life in Social Science & Clinical Medicine, 9(1).

Barcaccia, B. "Accepting limitations of life: leading our patients through a painful but healing path", invited lecture, Ludwig-Maximilians Universität, Munich, June, 10th 2008, Leopoldstr. 13 80802 München Department Psychologie.

Barcaccia B., Mismetti L., & Saliani A.M. (2010, October). Distress, Quality of Life and communication issues between oncological patients and significant others, Paper presented at the 40th Annual EABCT Congress, Milan, IT.

Beck, A.T. (1976). Cognitive therapy and the emotional disorders. New York: International Universities Press.

Benito-León, J., Rivera-Navarro, J., Guerrero, A.L., De Las Heras, V., Balseiro, J., Rodríguez, E., Belló, M., Martínez-Martín P. 2011. The CAREQOL-MS was a useful instrument to measure caregiver quality of life in multiple sclerosis. Journal of clinical epidemiology 64(6):675-86.

Berzon, R., Hays, R.D., Shumaker, S.A. (1993). International use, application, and performance of health-related quality of life instruments. Quality of Life Research 2:367–368.

Bowling, A. (1995). What things are important in people's lives? A survey of the public's judgements to inform scales of health related quality of life. Social Science & Medicine, 41: 1447-1462.

Bowling, A. (2001). Measuring disease: a review of disease-specific quality of life measurement scales (2nd ed.). Buckingham, U.K.: Open University Press.

Calman K. C. (1984). Quality of Life in Cancer Patients – An Hypothesis. Journal of Medical Ethics, 10, 124-127.

Cella, D. F. (1996). Quality of life outcomes: Measurement and validation. Oncology, 10 (Suppl 11), 233-246.

Chen, T. H., Li, L., & Kochen, M. M. (2005). A systematic review: How to choose appropriate health-related quality of life (HRQoL) measures in routine general practice? Journal of Zhejiang University Science, 6B(9), 936-940.

Ellis, A. (1994). Reason and emotion in psychotherapy: A comprehensive method of treating human disturbances (revised and updated). New York, NY: Carol Publishing.

Farquhar, M. 1995. Elderly people's definitions of quality of life. Social Science & Medicine 41: 1439-46.

Ferrans, C.E., Zerwic, J.J., Wilbur, J.E. & Larson, J.L. (2005). Conceptual model of health-related quality of life. Journal of Nursing Scholarship, 37, 336-342.

Gurková, E. (2011). Issues in the definitions of HRQoL. Journal of Nursing, Social Studies, Public Health and Rehabilitation 3–4, 190–197.

Lin, X.-J., Lin, I.M., Fan, S.-Y (2012). Methodological issues in measuring health-related quality of life, Tzu-Chi Medical Journal, in press, corrected proof, http://dx.doi.org/10.1016/j.tcmj.2012.09.002.

Malkina-Pykh, I.G., and Pykh,Y.A. 2008. Quality-of-life indicators at different scales: Theoretical background. Ecological Indicators 8: 854-62.

Marcos Del Cano, A.M. (2001). The concept of quality of life: Legal aspects. Medicine, Health Care and Philosophy 4: 91–95.

Martinez-Martin, P., and Kurtis, M.M. (2012). Health-related quality of life as an outcome variable in Parkinson's disease Therapeutic Advances in Neurological Disorders, 5(2): 105–117.

Mismetti L., & Barcaccia B. (2011, June). Anxiety, Depression, Quality of Life and communication issues in oncological patients and their informal caregivers, Paper presented at the 7th International Congress of Cognitive Psychotherapy, Istanbul, TR.

Pallini S., Bove G., & Laghi, F. (2011). Classification of professional values based on motivational content: an exploratory study on Italian Adolescents. Measurement and Evaluation in Counseling and Development, 44, 16-31.

Saliani A., Barcaccia B. & Mancini F. (2011). Interpersonal vicious cycles in Anxiety Disorders. In: Communication in Cognitive Behavioural Therapy, Rimondini M. (ed.). New York: Springer.

Segrin, C., Badger, T.A., Dorros, S.M., Meek, P., & Lopez, A.M. (2007). Interdependent anxiety and psychological distress in women with breast cancer and their partners. Psycho-Oncology, 16, 634-643.

Sheppard-Jones, Kathleen, "Quality of life dimensions for adults with developmental disabilities" (2003). University of Kentucky Doctoral Dissertations. Paper 335. http://uknowledge.uky.edu/gradschool_diss/335 (accessed December 1, 2012).

Testa, M.A., Simonson, D.C. (1996) Assessment of quality-of-life outcomes. New England Journal of Medicine 28:835–40.

Theofilou, P. (2012). Outcome Measurement in Palliative Care: Quality of Life. Journal of AIDS & Clinical Research, 3(5), 1-6.

Wasserman, D., Bickenbach, J. & Wachbroit, R. (2005). Introduction, In: D. Wasserman, J. Bickenbach & R. Wachbroit (eds.). Quality of Life and Human Difference: Genetic Testing, Health Care, and Disability (pp.1-26). New York: Cambridge University Press.

Wilson, I. (2004). The challenge of understanding articles about health-related quality of life. Clinical infectious diseases 39(3): 434-436.

Wilson, I. B., & Cleary, P. D. (1995). Linking clinical variables with health-related quality of life. A conceptual model of patient outcomes. Journal of the American Medical Association, 273(1), 59-65.

World Health Organisation Quality of Life Group (WHO). 1995. The World Health Organisation quality of life assessment (WHOQOL) position paper from the WHO. Social Science and Medicine 41: 347–52, 1403–09.

Ziller, R. C. (1974). Self-other orientation and quality of life. Social Indicators Research, 1,301–27.

CHAPTER 3

Assessing Health - Related Quality of Life in Chronic Kidney Disease Patients: The Use of General and Specific Instruments

Stefania S. Grigoriou[1,2], Christina Karatzaferi[1,2] and Giorgos K. Sakkas[1,2,*]

[1]*Department of Kinesiology, Center for Research and Technology, Hellas, Greece and* [2]*Department of Physical Education and Sport Science, University of Thessaly, Greece*

Abstract: Chronic kidney disease (CKD) has detrimental effects on patient's quality of life. Regarding this multidimensional concept, the correlations between assessment of quality of life, morbidity and mortality for this population indicate the measures' necessity. The Health Related Quality of Life (HRQoL) is a multidimensional approach that has been proposed as a way to achieve a more holistic assessment for the level of QoL in patients with CKD. Two dimensions have been included: the 'Generic' and the 'disease - targeted' multidimensional HRQoL questionnaires. Morever, selection criteria for the appropriate instrument are discussed identifying thus the utility of practicality, shortness and adaptability to CKD patients. This chapter provides specially the minimum requirements that any instrument of quality of life should meet in order to be functional in the everyday clinical practice. On the other hand, researchers in contrast to clinicians are focused mainly on generic or specific measures with high validity and reproducibility. Finally in this chapter, various interventions with proven effect in HRQoL are discussed, such as exercise and congitive behaviour therapy that may influence the psychosocial status in CKD patients affecting among others their daily function, the ability to sustain social networks and the overall mental and physical health.

Keywords: Renal, kidney, failure, survival, fatiguc, sleep, gender, illness, health - related quality of life, hemodialysis, renal failure, questionnaire, depression, mental health, exercise, cognitive behaviour therapy.

ASSESSING HRQoL

Quality of Life in CKD Patients

Quality of life (QoL) is a complex and multidimensional concept. It is well documented that patients with Chronic Kidney Disease (CKD) experience

*****Address correspondence to Giorgos K. Sakkas:** Department of Kinesiology, Center for Research and Technology Hellas, Institute of Research and Technology Thessaly, Karies, GR42100, Thessaly, Greece; Tel:+0030-2431-500-911; Fax: +0030-24310-69191; E-mail: gsakkas@med.uth.gr

Paraskevi Theofilou (Ed)

reduced levels of QoL compared to persons with other chronic illnesses (Loos, Briancon *et al.*, 2003). Even though the dialysis procedure is life-saving it is also a life-altering experience requiring a re-definition of a patient's overall life approach. The mental and physical state of their health often affects the perception of their QoL significantly suppressing the various roles that the person is called to play (Ugurlu, Bastug *et al.*, 2012).

Interestingly, after dialysis initiation, patients often shift their expectation from a "survival mode" to ways of improving the overall health status (Rettig and Sadler, 1997). Even though QoL in CKD patients is frequently overlooked, since other aspects of their general health are urgent matters, still a QoL score should be included in the patients' general health assessment since it correlates to hospitalization rates and mortality in this population (DeOreo, 1997). Understanding why QoL is important for a patient's survival and prognosis, will reveal QoL score to be a powerful tool in the hands of the health care providers for assessing non-traditional risk factors that might influence hospitalization and mortality rates and thus help patients delay their disease progression (Yen, Lin *et al.*, 2011). How a QoL score is measured will be explained later in this chapter.

Quality of Life as a Prognostic Factor in Patients with CKD

QoL is an important indicator of the overall health status but also reflects the patients' perception of the level of received care. Such perception could be used as an alternative tool for assessing the effectiveness of overall health care not only in renal disease patients but also in various chronic diseases. By assessing various aspects related to QoL, the health care providers could get additional information regarding the physical and mental perception of their patients' health (Kimmel, Emont *et al.*, 2003; Unruh, Benz *et al.*, 2004).

It is well known that QoL is a strong predictor of morbidity and mortality in patients with end - stage kidney disease (ESKD) especially in those with a high body mass index (Tsai, Hung *et al.*, 2010). In addition, the QoL score is a predictor of the patient's clinical condition and it is associated with prospective hospitalization (Lopes, Bragg-Gresham *et al.*, 2007), tendency to skip dialysis treatments and the possibility of depression (DeOreo, 1997). Previous research demonstrated that the functional status and the QoL score can early predict mortality among patients who enter dialysis treatment (McClellan, Anson *et al.*, 1991; Feroze, Noori *et al.*, 2011). The Dialysis Outcomes and Practice Patterns Study (DOPPS), a large, international observational study, demonstrated that three aspects of health related QoL - Physical Component Summary (PCS), Kidney Disease Component Summary (KDCS) and Mental Component Summary (MCS) - were associated with a higher risk of death and hospitalization in hemodialysis patients (Mapes, Lopes *et al.*, 2003). Finally, the QoL score could serve as an indicator of wellbeing since it is affected by the patients' perception of their overall health status (Kring and Crane, 2009).

TOOLS FOR ASSESSING QOL IN CKD

The Health Related Quality of Life (HRQOL) is a multidimensional approach that has been proposed as a way to achieve a more holistic assessment for the level of QoL in patients with CKD (Koller and Lorenz, 2002). Two dimensions have been included: the 'Generic' multidimensional HRQOL instruments for assessing the functionality and well-being of CKD patients and the 'disease-targeted' multidimensional HRQOL questionnaires for assessing characteristics common to a subgroup of the CKD patients.

Scales and Items for QoL

Most of the QoL questionnaires contain various questions (items) that are clustered together in groups (scales). The questions represent the items of the questionnaire which assess a single aspect of QoL (such as a physical symptom). However, since the concept of QoL is more complicated than a single item, very often the questionnaires contain a multi-item scale (group of items) combining several questions. Most instruments consist of a multi-item scale type of content (Fayers and Machin, 2007).

Constructs vs. Latent Variables

Construct and latent variables are in general abstract concepts. They describe some aspects that in general are not directly and reliably measurable while in some cases they describe the opinions of the investigator. Most of the times, construct and latent factors are used to describe aspects of QoL that are very difficult to distinguish and assess. For example, a latent variable is an item that assesses anxiety while a construct variable is the whole concept of QoL (Fayers and Machin, 2007).

Single vs. Multi item Scales

In a case of a latent trait or factor that influences the data, the approach of assessing the variable is described as being unidimensional (single). There is a possibility of some lower level factors, such as emotional functioning and cognitive functioning that are often described as being multidimensional and assessed as that (Fayers and Machin, 2007).

Psychometric vs. Clinimetric Scales

Psychometric strategies used in fields like psychology and education aim to develop one scale (or multiple scales) that measure single patient's characteristics or an underlying latent variable. Psychometric variables are useful because they help the assessment of variables that affect QoL and improve the communication between patients and health care providers. Regarding the reliability of those tools, the psychometric instrument presents internal consistency and stability without being influenced by the overall health status of the patient. About validity, the tool indicates characteristics such as construct, content, face, ecological, discriminant validity and responsiveness when QoL changes as a result of a strong stimulant. Finally, regarding the utility of the psychometric instruments, they can be found in many types of clinical research including cross-sectional and longitudinal study designs (Wright and Feinstein, 1992).

Clinimetric as a term was introduced by Feinstein in 1992 and represent an alternative approach, compared to the psychometric tools. Clinimetric strategies used in clinical medicine are based on the judgments of patients and clinicians and aim to assess clinical phenomena that are generally believed to comprise several unrelated patient characteristics or attributes. The documentation and characterization of a clinical phenomenon is the main goal of a clinimetrcic instrument (Wright and Feinstein, 1992).

Indicator vs. Causal Variables

Indicators describe variables that actually exist and are assumed to have some relationship to an underlying concept that the instrument tries to measure while the items do not alter or influence the underlying concept (Fayers and Hand, 2002). For example, a patient's perception of QoL or how aspects of their QoL status are impaired are indicators rather than items that cause impairment.

Causal variables on the other hand are variables which are part of the definition of what the concept being measured means and if they are present then the concept to be assessed is present. For example, the symptoms of a disease could have an adverse effect in QoL but they don't need to be present for low QoL. However if the symptom is present, then it is likely that the patients will have a low QoL score. This is a "causal variable" (Fayers and Machin, 2007).

Instruments for Assessing QoL

The assessment of QoL is divided into two general types: the generic and the disease specific as pretended in Table **1** (Theofilou, 2013).

Generic type – Quality of Life: A generic type of assessment is irrespective of condition or illness but the values resulting from this approach allow for comparisons between different groups of patients and interventions (Fayers and Machin, 2007). The generic type of assessment helps us evaluate health status across many different domains of the QoL. One of the most commonly used generic instrument for the assessment of the QoL is the **Short Form-36 Health Survey (SF-36)**. The SF-36 Item Short Form (Ware and Sherbourne, 1992) is a self-reported questionnaire and is composed of 36-items that measure eight health symptom dimensions. Those are: 1) Physical functioning (PF; is a ten-question scale that captures abilities to deal with the physical requirements of life, such as attending to personal needs, walking, and flexibility), 2) Role physical (RP; is a four-item scale that evaluates the extent to which physical capabilities limit activity), 3) Bodily pain (BP; bodily pain is a two-item scale that evaluates the perceived amount of pain experienced during the preceding 4 weeks and the extent to which that pain interfered with normal activities), 4) General health (GH; is a five-item scale that evaluates general health in terms of personal perception), 5) Vitality (VT; is a four-item scale that evaluates feelings of pep, 'energy' levels, and fatigue), 6) Social functioning (SF; is a two-item scale that evaluates the extent and amount of time, if any, that physical health or emotional problems interfered with family, friends, and other social interactions during the preceding 4 weeks), 7) Role Emotional (RE; is a three-item scale that evaluates the extent, if any, to which emotional factors interfere with work or other activities) and 8) Mental health (MH; is a five-item scale that evaluates feelings principally of anxiety and depression). In addition there is a single-item called Health Transition (HT) (five response categories ranging from "much better" to "much worse"), which is not used in scoring the scales or summary measures, but has been shown to be useful in estimating average changes in health status during the year prior to its administration. The eight health symptom dimensions are grouped into two domains components of health called the "Physical Component Summary" (PCS) and the "Mental Component Summary" (MCS) (Ware and Sherbourne, 1992).

The **WHOQOL-BREF** is an abbreviated generic Quality of Life Scale developed through the World Health Organization. It is composed of 26-item consisting of four domains (The WHOQOL GROUP, 1998): 1) physical health (mobility, daily activities, functional capacity, energy, pain, and sleep), 2) psychological health (self-image, negative thoughts, positive attitudes, self-esteem, mentality, learning ability, memory concentration, religion, and mental status), 3) social relationships (personal relationships, social support, and sex life), and 4) environmental health (financial resources, safety, health and social services, living physical environment, opportunities to acquire new skills and knowledge, recreation, general environment (noise, air pollution, *etc.*), and transportation). Moreover it includes items related to overall QoL and general health. Every item scores from 1 to 5 on a response scale, which is stipulated as a five-point ordinal scale. The scores are then transformed linearly to a 0–100-scale (Harper, Power *et al.*, 1998; Skevington and Tucker, 1999).

Another HRQOL tool is the **EuroQol 5-D** or **EQ-5D** of Brooks *et al.,* (1996). This instrument is short and contains five dimensions: 1) mobility, 2) self-care, 3) usual activities, 4) pain/discomfort, and 5) anxiety/depression. Every dimension has three response options: "no problems", "moderate problems", and "extreme problems". Therefore, it classifies a respondent's health status into one of 243 health states. The EQ–5D time trade-off scores range from 1 (full health) to –0.59 (0, being dead) (Brooks, 1996).

The **Sickness Impact Profile (SIP)** (Bergner, Bobbitt *et al.*, 1981) is a generic health status questionnaire that measures changes in the person's behavior as a consequence of illness on health-related QoL. This instrument measures dysfunction and contains 136 items grouped into 12 domains: 1) sleep and rest, 2) emotional behavior, 3) body care and movement, 4) home management, 5) mobility, 6) social interaction, 7) ambulation, 8) alertness behavior, 9) communication, 10) work, 11) eating, and 12) recreation and pastimes. The higher the scores on the SIP, the more severe is the disability.

The **Missoula-Vitas Quality of Life Index** (**MVQOLI**) is an instrument that assess the qualitative and subjective experience of QoL in a way that can be quickly interpreted by professional caregivers (Byock and Merriman 1998). The questionnaire contains 26 items, one global QoL item and covers 5 aspects of the QoL: 1) disease symptoms, 2) function, 3) interpersonal, 4) wellbeing and 5) transcendence (Namisango, Katabira *et al.,* 2007). The MVQOLI has two versions: the short 15-item and long 25-item. The initial instrument was the long version with the 25 items however it was considered very long for patients and therefore it was reduced down to the 15-item version which is actually the most used (Theofilou, Kapsalis & Panagiotaki, 2012; Theofilou, Aroni, Ralli, Gouza & Zyga, 2013a).

The **Schedule for the Evaluation of Individual Quality of Life - SEIQoL** is a semi-structured two-part instrument. On the first part, the users have to name five cues or life areas and then marks on a bar chart their perceived position, in terms of either best or worst possible satisfaction. This yields five scores, ranging from 0 to 100, which are termed the cue levels. The second part consists of a disk containing five independently moveable or overlapping disks, each of which represents different aspects of the QoL. The user determines the relative importance, or 'weight', of each life area chosen, by manipulating the circular disks. The tool can be applied in its entirety in approximately 15 minutes (O'Boyle, Browne *et al.*, 1993).

A preference-based measurement of quality of life could be achieved by the **Quality of Well-Being Self-Administered** version (**QWB-SA**) (Kaplan, Sieber *et al.*, 1997) which is derived from the longer, more complex, and less functional

Quality of Well-Being Scale (QWB) (Kaplan and Anderson, 1988). The QWB-SA questionnaire consists of 76-items and assesses the level of functioning in mobility, physical activity, and social activity as well as 58 acute and chronic symptoms. Reliability and validity levels of the QWB-SA are similar to the original QWB.

The **Illness Effects Questionnaire (IEQ)** contains 20 short items to assess HRQOL. The questionnaire evaluates the patient's perception regarding the effect of their disease on their quality of life (Peterson and Greenberg, 1989). Especially, it evaluates the extent to which the disease affects the patients' lives in a scale from 0 to 7 and whether the patients disagree (0 to 3) or agree (4 to 7) with its content. The higher the score the higher distress the person experiences.

Disease-specific - Chronic Kidney Disease: One of the first subjective self-report questionnaires that measure QoL in CKD patients was the **Quality of Life Index – Dialysis Version III (QLI-D)** including 34 pairs of questions (Ferrans and Powers, 1985). The questionnaire assesses health care, physical health and functioning, occupation, education, leisure, the future, peace of mind, personal faith, life goals, personal appearance, self-acceptance, general happiness, and general satisfaction. In addition the QLI-D assesses two additional variables related to potential changes due to renal failure and the possibility of kidney transplantation could affect patients' perceived QoL.

The **Kidney Disease Quality of Life Short Form (KDQOL-SF)** version is a shorter version of the original Kidney Disease Quality of Life questionnaire (Hays, Kallich *et al.*, 1997). It's a self-report questionnaire designed for chronic kidney disease patients and those on dialysis. The instrument consists of 36 general health items and 43 kidney-specific items. The general health items are divided mainly between physical and mental health across eight sub-scales: 1) Physical functioning, 2) Role physical, 3) Pain, 4) General health, 5) Emotional well-being, 6) Role emotional, 7) Social function and 8) Energy/fatigue. The 43 kidney-specific items assess the particular effects of the disease in activities of daily living, work status, and social interaction. Finally, the measurement includes one overall health rating item ranging from 0 ("worst possible health") to 10 ("best possible health."). The 80 items take about 16 minutes to complete.

The **Choices Health Experience Questionnaire (CHEQ)** is a disease specific instrument designed to assess HRQoL while it takes into account information such as dialysis modality and dialysis dose (Wu, Fink *et al.*, 2001). The questionnaire includes 83 items and consists of two parts: The first part contains 9 general domains from the SF-36 questionnaire (physical function, role-physical, bodily pain, mental health, role-emotional, social function, vitality, general health, and report transition) while the second part consists of 16 dialysis specific domains (role-physical, mental health, general health, freedom, travel restriction, cognitive function, financial function, restriction diet and fluids, recreation, work, body image, symptoms, sex, sleep, access, and quality of life) (Wu, Fink *et al.*, 2001).

The **Renal Quality of Life Profile (RQLP)** instrument is a specific and self-administered questionnaire (Salek, 1999). The 43-itemed questionnaire is grouped into 5 dimensions: Eating and drinking, physical activities, leisure time, psychosocial activities and impact of treatment. It has shown good validity and reliability and has successfully tested in a recent clinical study in diabetic patients (Salek & Reakes, 1994).

The **Renal-Dependent Individualized Quality of life Questionnaire** (Bradley, 1997) was developed out of a diabetes-specific individualized quality of life questionnaire, the Audit of Diabetes Dependent Quality of Life (ADDQoL) (Bradley, Todd *et al.*, 1999). The specific questionnaire assesses the chronic renal failure patients' perception of quality of life. This instrument, like the RQLP, has been studied in clinical research trials. Future research will indicate the usefulness and acceptance of these assessments to evaluate the quality of life in patients with CKD and whether their results will lead to therapeutic interventions.

Table 1: QoL Instruments.

Name	Instrument	References	Validity	Reliability
Short Form-36 Health Survey (SF-36)	Generic	(Ware & Sherbourne, 1992)	None reported Convergent (Mingardi, Cornalba *et al.*, 1999) Content and construct (Sigstad, Stray-Pedersen *et al.*, 2005)	For physical components = 0.91 and 0.88 for the mental components

Table 1: contd…

WHOQOL-BREF	Generic	(1998) (Niu and Li 2005)	None reported None reported	None reported a = 0.69 for all scales a= 0.93 for whole scales
EuroQol 5-D or EQ-5D	Generic	(Brooks *et al.*, 1996)	None reported	0.90
Sickness Impact Profile (SIP)	Generic	(Bergner, Bobbit *et al.*, 1981)	Convergent and discriminant validity	test-retest reliability (r = 0.92)
Missoula-Vitas Quality of Life Index (MVQOLI)	Generic	(Byock and Merriman 1998)	0.43	0.77
Schedule for the Evaluation of Individual Quality of Life- SEIQoL	Generic	(O' Boyle, Browne *et al.*, 1993)	0.49 - 0.74	None reported
Quality of Well-Being Self-Administered (QWB-SA)	Generic	(Kaplan, Sieber *et al.*, 1997)	None reported	None reported
Illness Effects Questionnaire (IEQ)	Generic	(Peterson & Greenberg, 1989)	None reported	None reported
Quality of Life Index – Dialysis Version III (QLI-D)	Disease-specific	(Ferrans & Powers, 1985)	The correlation between the QLI-D and life satisfaction was 0.65	0.88 - 0.93
Kidney Disease Quality of Life Short Form (KDQOL-SF)	Disease-specific	(Hays, Kallich, Jet *et al.*, 1997) (Bakewell, Higgins *et al.,* 2001)	None reported Non reported	0.68 to 0.94 a>0.70 for each domain except sleep
Choices Health Experience Questionnaire (CHEQ)	Disease-specific	(Wu, Fink *et al.*, 2001)	Convergent and discriminant construct validity	For scales greater than 0.70 and overall QOL (0.68) r= 0.55 to 0.79
Renal Quality of Life Profile (RQLP)	Disease-specific	(Salek, 1999)	Face and content validity	None reported
Renal-dependent individualized quality of life questionnaire	Disease-specific	(Bradley 1997)	Face and content validity	None reported

Administration of Questionnaires – Interview Modality

It is very important to denote that the administration of a questionnaire has to follow some particular rules especially when sensitive populations like the CKD or ESKD patients are used. The ability to interview is a skill. The interview as a methodological approach is useful for getting all the related information behind the patient's experience where depth of meaning is important. In general it is assumed that the interviewer should be familiar with the topic, tolerant and sensitive and not biased toward the study's outcome. An interview can be structured or semi-structured. The 'structured' interview is similar to type of questionnaire using closed questions while the 'semi-structured' interview involves many open-ended questions, although they may also contain some closed type questions (Gomm, 2004).

SELECTION CRITERIA FOR THE APPROPRIATE INSTRUMENT

There is wide interest from researchers to develop instruments that will be applicable to the daily clinical practice by the health care providers. It is very important for the patients that the assessment of QoL becomes part of the everyday clinical practice and part of the routine examination but also very important for the clinician to feel comfortable with the assessment tools and with the meaning of the final scores. In contrast to clinicians, researchers are focused on generic or specific measures with high validity and reproducibility rather than the applicability and usefulness. Overall, the instruments for assessing QoL, either generic or disease specific should be practical, short, adaptable and easy to answer and administer to the patient (Doward, Meads *et al.*, 2004).

Clinical Focus

Any instrument should meet at least some minimum requirements in order to be used in the clinical setting. Failure on some of those requirements could affect the way data are being analyzed and interpreted as well as the final conclusions made from the assessment.

Any scale should be *unidimensional* in order to provide high validity scores. Also *reliability* is necessary in order to secure at the scale could get the same score on repeated uses under the same conditions (Bardsley and Coles, 1992). *Construct validity,* which refers to whether a scale measures or correlates with the theorized psychological scientific construct that it purports to measure, is very important in order to assess the majority of the aspects related to the QoL (Hunt, McEwen *et al.,* 1986). *Face and content validity* is useful for checking the content of the instrument including aspects related to the patients' level of understanding and easiness to complete it (Hunt and McKenna, 1992). *Sensitivity of change* confirms that the instrument can detect changes over time before and after an intervention (Ware, Rogers *et al.,* 1986). Any measure should meet *appropriateness* standards and to be applicable to patients. Finally it is important for any instrument to meet *practicability* standards. That means that a measure is practical for use in clinical practice when accurate information about patients, treatments and outcomes is included (Cox, Fitzpatrick *et al.,* 1992).

Research Focus

According to Fayer & Machin (2007) the evaluating criteria for a research study are the following:

1) Clear conceptual and measurement model,

2) Reliability is the degree to which an instrument is free from random error,

3) Validity refers to the degree to which the instrument measures what it is designed to measure,

4) *Responsiveness* is an instrument's ability to detect change overtime,

5) *Interpretability* is defined as the degree to which one can assign qualitative meaning, that is, clinical or commonly understood connotations, to quantitative scores,

6) Respondent and administrative burden refer to the time, effort, and other demands placed on those to whom the instrument is administered (respondent burden) or on those who administer the instrument (administrative burden),

7) *Alternative forms* refer to all the ways that an instrument might be administered other than the original way,

8) *Cultural and language adaptations* (translations)- the equivalence is necessary between the original instrument and its adaptation (Lohr, Aaronson *et al.,* 1996),

9) *Sensitivity* is the ability of instrument to detect the differences between groups and patients.

INTERVENTIONS IMPROVING QOL IN CKD

Research has pointed out that many factors influence the QoL levels in CKD including socio-demographic and disease specific. Gender is one of the most common characteristics affecting QoL, with females reporting worse HRQoL than men (Rocco, Gassman *et al.*, 1997; Jofre, Lopez-Gomez *et al.*, 1998; Mingardi, Cornalba *et al.*, 1999). The cause is often the increased prevalence of depression as well as the higher frequency of negative perception of the disease among female patients. In addition to gender, low social status and education, as well as lack of employment correlated highly with decreased QoL (Simmons and Abress, 1990; Rocco, Gassman *et al.*, 1997).

The *stage of the disease* is one of the most common factors affecting QoL with the event of renal transplantation to be the best treatment option for improving QoL in people with end stage renal disease (Wyld, Morton *et al.*, 2012). Comparing the various replacement modalities, studies have shown that peritoneal dialysis achieves higher scores in HRQoL compared to traditional hemodialysis therapy (Diaz-Buxo, Lowrie *et al.*, 2000).

It well documented that the *renal failure per se*, independently of comorbid conditions, affect the levels of QoL in patients with CKD (Van Manen, Korevaar *et al.*, 2003; Barotfi, Molnar *et al.*, 2006). Regarding comorbidity, congestive heart failure and anemia predict low QoL (Silverberg, Wexler *et al.*, 2005). In studies aiming to improve HRQoL, researchers have targeted the level of hemoglobin values by the administration of erythropoiesis stimulating agents and have found a significant effect in social functioning and mental health domains but lower improvements in aspects related to emotional functioning and pain (Leaf and Goldfarb, 2009).

Psychosocial factors can also predict HRQoL scores. Depression, in particular, is one of the most common factors that affect the daily function, the patients' ability to sustain social networks, and as it is expected their QoL (Kutner, 2008). Regarding in particular peritoneal dialysis patients, depression and low QoL correlated with higher comorbidity, poorer nutritional status, anemia and increased hospitalization rates (Lew and Piraino, 2005). Theofilou *et al.,* (2010) found that hemodialysis patients with many years in dialysis showed decreased levels of QoL, while they experienced deterioration in physical, social and environmental health. In contrast the peritoneal dialysis patients did not show any link between duration of therapy and levels of QoL (Theofilou and Panagiotaki, 2010). Other psychosocial factor such as anxiety, fear of allograft rejection, loss of control, body image, sexual problems, social support, and unemployment influence significantly HRQoL in CKD patients as well (Mucsi, 2008). Even though most of these factors are modifiable by various interventions (including exercise, see below), still little research has been done in improving QoL in CKD patients.

Studies using *Cognitive Behavior Therapy* (CBT) through interventions targeting educational status, cognitive function and behavior have shown enhanced adherence to one of the most challenging for hemodialysis patients restrictions - the one of the fluids' intake restriction (Sharp, Wild *et al.*, 2005). Cognitive-behavioral intervention can improve the psychosocial status in CKD patients affecting domains such as general health status, social functioning, burden of kidney disease, depressed mood, anxiety, and mastery (Weiner, Kutner *et al.*, 2010). Reviewing the literature, a recent study by Hedayati *et al.,* (2012) indicated that the CBT approach seems to be very promising in enhancing QoL in CKD patients while it is feasible to take place in nephrology departments and dialysis units (Hedayati, Yalamanchili *et al.*, 2012). According to a recent study conducted by Abraham *et al.,* (2012) applied counseling in patients with ESKD resulted in improvements in the psychological domain and changes in awareness were reported, while there was evidence of improvements in patients' misconception about their disease. Patients that followed counseling interventions increased their positive feelings, concentration level, thinking and learning power (Abraham, Venu *et al.*, 2012).

Researchers suggest that the CBT approach could improve sleep quality which is one of the most prominent issues for the CKD patients, its disturbance leading to low perceived QoL and affecting overall health (Gusbeth-Tatomir, Boisteanu *et al.*, 2007; Elder, Pisoni *et al.*, 2008).

Efficient management of sleep disorders could be thus beneficial in improving CKD patients' QoL. Contributing factors to disturbed sleep include conditions such as restless legs syndrome, periodic leg movements during sleep, sleep apnea, insomnia and depression (Hopkins 2005; Sakkas, Gourgoulianis *et al.*, 2008). In the case of restless legs, intradialytic exercise has been shown to improve severity of symptoms and QoL in ESKD patients with RLS (Sakkas, Hadjigeorgiou *et al.*, 2008). Recent studies have shown that the pineal hormone melatonin could be used to treat sleep disorders in these patients population (Russcher, Koch *et al.*, 2012). The influence of melatonin in circadian sleep-wake rhythm is proven to be beneficial since it can regulate the circadian sleep-wake rhythm improving furthermore the QoL in these patients (Koch, Nagtegaal *et al.*, 2010; Russcher, Koch *et al.*, 2012).

Another very important factor that influences QoL in CKD patients is the levels of physical activity. The majority of the CKD patients are physically inactive and they have serious difficulties in completing their daily activities and this is often translated as a low health related quality QoL (Johansen, Chertow *et al.*, 2000; Padilla, Krasnoff *et al.*, 2008). In addition, the sedentary life style adopted by these patients imposes a systematic effect on their general health increasing significantly the risk of a cardiovascular episode (Green, O'Driscoll *et al.*, 2008). It is well documented that regular exercise decreases the risk of mortality and improves the QoL in both dialysis (Thompson, Buchner *et al.*, 2003; Petrella, Lattanzio *et al.*, 2005) and pre dialysis CKD patients (Mustata, Groeneveld *et al.*, 2011). There is a causal relationship between exercise and QoL, where implementation of an exercise training programme in patients receiving hemodialysis therapy can improve the physiological, psychological, and functional aspects of an individual's life (Sakkas, Sargeant *et al.*, 2003; Sakkas, 2007; Takhreem, 2008).

Kouidi *et al.,* (Kouidi, Iacovides *et al.,* 1997) also reported a 35% improvement in depression after 6 months of non-dialysis' days aerobic exercise in 20 patients. An improvement in depression symptoms (P=0.06) was observed in the study of Suh *et al.,* (Suh, Jung *et al.,* 2002) who assessed the influence of a 3-month aerobic training in 14 HD patients, with a parallel improvement in anxiety symptoms and QoL levels. Likewise, Malagoni *et al.,* (Malagoni, Catizone *et al.,* 2008) who examined the impact of a 6 month home-based exercise programme observed that the mental health (MH) scale of the SF-36 questionnaire improved significantly by about 30% at the end of the training period. In the study of Matsumoto *et al.,* (Matsumoto, Furuta *et al.,* 2007), the MH scale of the SF36 questionnaire was also found to be significantly improved after 12 months of aerobic exercise (by 8%). Reboredo *et al.,* (Reboredo Mde, Henrique *et al.,* 2010) found a 18% improvement in the MH scale of SF36 after a six-month intradialytic exercise training program. Moreover Cheema *et al.,* (Cheema, Abas *et al.,* 2007) examined the influence of a 3 months high-intensity intradialytic resistance training in depression, QoL and other factors related to muscle quality and quantity. Taking all into account, aerobic exercise training appeared to be an effective approach in terms of improving depression symptoms in HD patients, while could in parallel improve many aspects of the patient's health and wellbeing, resulting to an overall improvement in perceived QoL.

CONCLUSIONS

Chronic Kidney Disease patients exhibit low QoL levels, usually accompanied by significant emotional distress (Finkelstein, Wuerth *et al.,* 2009). A strong contributor to the low QoL levels is the hemodialysis treatment *per se*, which requires from the patient to stay attached to the dialysis machine for approximately 4 hours, 3 times a week, a fact that significantly restricts patient's independence (Theofilou, 2012a). There is a wide variety of health related QoL tools that can be used in CKD patients by health care providers however, many times, practical limitations and lack of knowledge impedes their usage in the majority of the clinical settings (Kalantar-Zadeh and Unruh, 2005).

Quality of life is a very important aspect of the overall health status and can be measured easily and very accurately by many questionnaires. A score of QoL is a useful tool in the hands of the health care providers that can help them to evaluate the overall quality of the care provided to their patients (Unruh and Hess, 2007). By improving sleep and treating depression and other psychiatric disorders, clinicians can dramatically improve patients' QoL and reduce overall mortality rate (Kimmel, 2005; Mucsi, Molnar *et al.*, 2005). Among other interventions, an increase in levels of physical activity by organized exercise training programs (during hemodialysis or home based) could reduce factors that negatively affect QoL such as depression and boredom, while it could positively influence other factors such as self-esteem, body image and functionality that improve patients' QoL. Assessment of the quality of life should be incorporated in the routine examination of all CKD patients and should be re-evaluated very often in order to monitor patients' experiences and perceptions as well as gauge the quality of patient's care and overall support.

ACKNOWLEDGEMENT

None Declared.

CONFLICT OF INTEREST

None Declared.

REFERENCES

Abraham, S., A. Venu, *et al.,* (2012). Assessment of quality of life in patients on hemodialysis and the impact of counseling. Saudi J Kidney Dis Transpl 23(5): 953-957.

Bakewell, A. B., R. M. Higgins, *et al.,* (2001). Does ethnicity influence perceived quality of life of patients on dialysis and following renal transplant? Nephrology Dialysis Transplantation 16(7): 1395-1401.

Bardsley, M. J. and J. M. Coles (1992). Practical experiences in auditing patient outcomes. Qual Health Care 1(2): 124-130.

Barotfi, S., M. Z. Molnar, *et al.,* (2006). Validation of the Kidney Disease Quality of Life-Short Form questionnaire in kidney transplant patients. Journal of Psychosomatic Research 60(5): 495-504.

Bergner, M., R. A. Bobbitt, *et al.,* (1981). The Sickness Impact Profile: development and final revision of a health status measure. Med Care 19(8): 787-805.

Bradley, C. (1997). Design of a renal-dependent individualized quality of life questionnaire. Adv Perit Dial 13: 116-120.

Bradley, C., C. Todd, *et al.,* (1999). The development of an individualized questionnaire measure of perceived impact of diabetes on quality of life: the ADDQoL. Quality of Life Research 8(1-2): 79-91.

Brooks, R. (1996). EuroQol: the current state of play. Health Policy 37(1): 53-72.

Byock, I. R. and M. P. Merriman (1998). Measuring quality of life for patients with terminal illness: the Missoula-VITAS (R) quality of life index. Palliative Medicine 12(4): 231-244.

Cheema, B., H. Abas, *et al.*, (2007). Progressive exercise for anabolism in kidney disease (PEAK): a randomized, controlled trial of resistance training during hemodialysis. J Am Soc Nephrol 18(5): 1594-1601.

Cox, D. R., R. Fitzpatrick, *et al.*, (1992). Quality-of-Life Assessment - Can We Keep It Simple. Journal of the Royal Statistical Society Series a-Statistics in Society 155: 353-393.

DeOreo, P. B. (1997). Hemodialysis patient-assessed functional health status predicts continued survival, hospitalization, and dialysis-attendance compliance. Am J Kidney Dis 30(2): 204-212.

Diaz-Buxo, J. A., E. G. Lowrie, *et al.*, (2000). Quality-of-life evaluation using short form 36: Comparison in hemodialysis and peritoneal dialysis patients. American Journal of Kidney Diseases 35(2): 293-300.

Doward, L. C., D. M. Meads, *et al.*, (2004). Requirements for quality of life instruments in clinical research. Value in Health 7 Suppl 1: S13-16.

Elder, S. J., R. L. Pisoni, *et al.*, (2008). Sleep quality predicts quality of life and mortality risk in haemodialysis patients: results from the Dialysis Outcomes and Practice Patterns Study (DOPPS). Nephrol Dial Transplant 23(3): 998-1004.

Fayers, P. and D. Machin (2007). Quality of life: The assessment, analysis and interpretation of patient-reported outcomes. 2nd Ed. Chichester. UK, John Wiley and Sons.

Fayers, P. M. and D. J. Hand (2002). Causual variables, indicator variables and measurements scales: an example from quality of life. Journal of Royal Statistical Society: Series A (Statistics in Society) 165(2): 233-261.

Feroze, U., N. Noori, *et al.*, (2011). Quality-of-life and mortality in hemodialysis patients: roles of race and nutritional status. Clin J Am Soc Nephrol 6(5): 1100-1111.

Ferrans, C. E. and M. J. Powers (1985). Quality of life index: development and psychometric properties. ANS Adv Nurs Sci 8(1): 15-24.

Finkelstein, F. O., D. Wuerth, *et al.*, (2009). Health related quality of life and the CKD patient: challenges for the nephrology community. Kidney Int 76(9): 946-952.

Gomm, R. (2004). Social research methodology : a critical introduction. Houndmills, Basingstoke, Hampshire ; New York, Palgrave Macmillan.

Green, D. J., G. O'Driscoll, *et al.*, (2008). Exercise and cardiovascular risk reduction: time to update the rationale for exercise? J Appl Physiol 105(2): 766-768.

Gusbeth-Tatomir, P., D. Boisteanu, *et al.*, (2007). Sleep disorders: a systematic review of an emerging major clinical issue in renal patients. Int Urol Nephrol 39(4): 1217-1226.

Harper, A., M. Power, *et al.*, (1998). Development of the World Health Organization WHOQOL-BREF quality of life assessment. Psychological Medicine 28(3): 551-558.

Hays RD, Kallich J, *et al.*, (1997). Kidney Disease Quality of Life Short Form (KDQOL-SF™) Version 1.3: A Manual for Use and Scoring. P-7994. Santa Monica, CA: Rand.

Hedayati, S. S., V. Yalamanchili, *et al.*, (2012). A practical approach to the treatment of depression in patients with chronic kidney disease and end-stage renal disease. Kidney International 81(3): 247-255.

Hopkins, K. (2005). Facilitating sleep for patients with end stage renal disease. Nephrol Nurs J 32(2): 189-190, 192-185.

Hunt, S. M., J. McEwen, *et al.,* (1986). Measuring health status. London ; Dover, N.H., Croom Helm.

Hunt, S. M. and S. P. McKenna (1992). The QLDS: a scale for the measurement of quality of life in depression. Health Policy 22(3): 307-319.

Jofre, R., J. M. Lopez-Gomez, *et al.,* (1998). Changes in quality of life after renal transplantation. American Journal of Kidney Diseases 32(1): 93-100.

Johansen, K. L., G. M. Chertow, *et al.,* (2000). Physical activity levels in patients on hemodialysis and healthy sedentary controls. Kidney International 57(6): 2564-2570.

Kalantar-Zadeh, K. and M. Unruh (2005). Health related quality of life in patients with chronic kidney disease. Int Urol Nephrol 37(2): 367-378.

Kaplan, R. M. and J. P. Anderson (1988). A general health policy model: update and applications. Health Serv Res 23(2): 203-235.

Kaplan, R. M., W. J. Sieber, *et al.,* (1997). The Quality of Well-Being Scale: Comparison of the interviewer-administered version with a self-administered questionnaire. Psychology & Health 12(6): 783-791.

Kimmel, P. L. (2005). Psychosocial factors in chronic kidney disease patients. Semin Dial 18(2): 71-72.

Kimmel, P. L., S. L. Emont, *et al.,* (2003). ESRD patient quality of life: Symptoms, spiritual beliefs, psychosocial factors, and ethnicity. American Journal of Kidney Diseases 42(4): 713-721.

Koch, B. C., J. E. Nagtegaal, *et al.,* (2010). Different melatonin rhythms and sleep-wake rhythms in patients on peritoneal dialysis, daytime hemodialysis and nocturnal hemodialysis. Sleep Med 11(3): 242-246.

Koller, M. and W. Lorenz (2002). Quality of life: a deconstruction for clinicians. Journal of the Royal Society of Medicine 95(10): 481-488.

Kouidi, E., A. Iacovides, *et al.,* (1997). Exercise renal rehabilitation program: psychosocial effects. Nephron 77(2): 152-158.

Kring, D. L. and P. B. Crane (2009). Factors affecting quality of life in persons on hemodialysis. Nephrol Nurs J 36(1): 15-24, 55.

Kutner, N. G. (2008). Promoting functioning and well-being in older CKD patients: review of recent evidence. Int Urol Nephrol 40(4): 1151-1158.

Leaf, D. E. and D. S. Goldfarb (2009). Interpretation and review of health-related quality of life data in CKD patients receiving treatment for anemia. Kidney International 75(1): 15-24.

Lew, S. Q. and B. Piraino (2005). Quality of life and psychological issues in peritoneal dialysis patients. Semin Dial 18(2): 119-123.

Lohr, K. N., N. K. Aaronson, *et al.,* (1996). Evaluating quality-of-life and health status instruments: development of scientific review criteria. Clin Ther 18(5): 979-992.

Loos, C., S. Briancon, *et al.,* (2003). Effect of end-stage renal disease on the quality of life of older patients. J Am Geriatr Soc 51(2): 229-233.

Lopes, A. A., J. L. Bragg-Gresham, *et al.,* (2007). Factors associated with health-related quality of life among hemodialysis patients in the DOPPS. Quality of Life Research 16(6): 1095-1095.

Malagoni, A. M., L. Catizone, *et al.,* (2008). Acute and long-term effects of an exercise program for dialysis patients prescribed in hospital and performed at home. J Nephrol 21(6): 871-878.

Mapes, D. L., A. A. Lopes, *et al.,* (2003). Health-related quality of life as a predictor of mortality and hospitalization: The Dialysis Outcomes and Practice Patterns Study (DOPPS). Kidney International 64(1): 339-349.

Matsumoto, Y., A. Furuta, *et al.,* (2007). The impact of pre-dialytic endurance training on nutritional status and quality of life in stable hemodialysis patients (Sawada study). Ren Fail 29(5): 587-593.

McClellan, W. M., C. Anson, *et al.,* (1991). Functional status and quality of life: predictors of early mortality among patients entering treatment for end stage renal disease. J Clin Epidemiol 44(1): 83-89.

Mingardi, G., L. Cornalba, *et al.,* (1999). Health-related quality of life in dialysis patients. A report from an Italian study using the SF-36 Health Survey. Nephrology Dialysis Transplantation 14(6): 1503-1510.

Mucsi, I. (2008). Health-Related Quality of Life in Chronic Kidney Disease Patients. Primary Psychiatry 15(1): 146-151.

Mucsi, I., M. Z. Molnar, *et al.,* (2005). Restless legs syndrome, insomnia and quality of life in patients on maintenance dialysis. Nephrol Dial Transplant 20(3): 571-577.

Mustata, S., S. Groeneveld, *et al.,* (2011). Effects of exercise training on physical impairment, arterial stiffness and health-related quality of life in patients with chronic kidney disease: a pilot study. Int Urol Nephrol 43(4): 1133-1141.

Namisango, E., E. Katabira, *et al.,* (2007). Validation of the Missoula-Vitas Quality-of-Life Index among patients with advanced AIDS in urban Kampala, Uganda. Journal of Pain and Symptom Management 33(2): 189-202.

Niu, S. F. and I. C. Li (2005). Quality of life of patients having renal replacement therapy. Journal of Advanced Nursing 51(1): 15-21.

O'Boyle, C., J. Browne, *et al.,* (1993). Schedule for the Evaluation of Individual Quality of Life (SEIQoL): A Direct Weighting Procedure for Quality of Life Domains (SEIQoL-DW). Dublin, Department of Psychology, Royal College of Surgeons, Administration Manual.

Padilla, J., J. Krasnoff, *et al.,* (2008). Physical functioning in patients with chronic kidney disease. J Nephrol 21(4): 550-559.

Peterson, R. and G. Greenberg (1989). The role of perception of illness. Health Psychologist 11: 2-3.

Petrella, R. J., C. N. Lattanzio, *et al.,* (2005). Can adoption of regular exercise later in life prevent metabolic risk for cardiovascular disease? Diabetes Care 28(3): 694-701.

Reboredo Mde, M., D. M. Henrique, *et al.,* (2010). Exercise training during hemodialysis reduces blood pressure and increases physical functioning and quality of life. Artif Organs 34(7): 586-593.

Rettig, R. A. and J. H. Sadler (1997). Measuring and improving the health status of end stage renal disease patients. Health Care Financ Rev 18(4): 77-82.

Rocco, M. V., J. J. Gassman, *et al.,* (1997). Cross-sectional study of quality of life and symptoms in chronic renal disease patients: The modification of diet in renal disease study. American Journal of Kidney Diseases 29(6): 888-896.

Russcher, M., B. Koch, *et al.,* (2012). The role of melatonin treatment in chronic kidney disease. Front Biosci 17: 2644-2656.

Sakkas, G. K., K. I. Gourgoulianis, *et al.,* (2008). Haemodialysis patients with sleep apnoea syndrome experience increased central adiposity and altered muscular composition and functionality. Nephrol Dial Transplant 23(1): 336-344.

Sakkas, G. K., G. M. Hadjigeorgiou, *et al.,* (2008). Intradialytic aerobic exercise training ameliorates symptoms of restless legs syndrome and improves functional capacity in patients on hemodialysis: a pilot study. Asaio J 54(2): 185-190.

Sakkas, G. K., Karatzaferi, C., Giannaki, C.D., Lavdas, E., Atmatzidis, E., Kanaki, A., Liakopoulos, V., Koutedakis, Y., Stefanids, I (2007). Aerobic exercise training improves sleep efficiency and reduces apnea episodes in hemodialysis patients. 40th American Society of Nephrology, October 31- November 5, 2007 San Francisco, California, USA, J Am Soc Nephrol. 18:485A.

Sakkas, G. K., A. J. Sargeant, *et al.,* (2003). Changes in muscle morphology in dialysis patients after 6 months of aerobic exercise training. Nephrol Dial Transplant 18(9): 1854-1861.

Salek, M. (1999). Quality of life in patients with end-stage renal disease. Journal of Applied Therapeutic Research 2(3): 163-170.

Salek, M. and A. Reakes (1994). Quality of life assessment in end-stage renal disease using a renal specific quality profile (RQLP): A practicality and validation study, Report I. University of Wales, Cardiff.

Sharp, J., M. R. Wild, *et al.,* (2005). A cognitive behavioral group approach to enhance adherence to hemodialysis fluid restrictions: a randomized controlled trial. Am J Kidney Dis 45(6): 1046-1057.

Sigstad, H. M., A. Stray-Pedersen, *et al.,* (2005). "Coping, quality of life, and hope in adults with primary antibody deficiencies." Health Qual Life Outcomes 3: 31.

Silverberg, D. S., D. Wexler, *et al.,* (2005). Effects of treatment with epoetin beta on outcomes in patients with anaemia and chronic heart failure. Kidney Blood Press Res 28(1): 41-47.

Simmons, R. G. and L. Abress (1990). Quality-of-life issues for end-stage renal disease patients. Am J Kidney Dis 15(3): 201-208.

Skevington, S. M. and C. Tucker (1999). Designing response scales for cross-cultural use in health care: Data from the development of the UK WHOQOL. British Journal of Medical Psychology 72: 51-61.

Suh, M. R., H. H. Jung, *et al.,* (2002). Effects of regular exercise on anxiety, depression, and quality of life in maintenance hemodialysis patients. Ren Fail 24(3): 337-345.

Takhreem, M. (2008). The effectiveness of intradialytic exercise prescription on quality of life in patients with chronic kidney disease. Medscape J Med 10(10): 226.

The WHOQOL GROUP (1998). The World Health Organization Quality of Life Assessment (WHOQOL): development and general psychometric properties. Soc Sci Med 46(12): 1569-1585.

Theofilou, P. (2013). Quality of life: Definition and Measurement. Europe's Journal of Psychology, 9: 150-162.

Theofilou, P., Aroni, A., Ralli, M., Gouzou, M., Zyga S. (2013a). Measuring health - related quality of life in haemodialysis patients: Psychometric properties of the Missoula-VITAS Quality of Life Index (MVQOLI-15) in Greece. Health Psychology Research, in press.

Theofilou, P, Kapsalis, F, Panagiotaki, H. (2012). Greek version of MVQOLI - 15: Translation and cultural adaptation. International Journal of Caring Sciences, 5(3), 289-294.

Theofilou, P. and H. Panagiotaki (2010). Quality of Life in Patients with Chronic Renal Failure: Differences between the Early and Later Years of Current Treatment. Nosileftiki 49(3): 295-304.

Theofilou, P. (2012a). Association of insomnia with kidney disease quality of life reported by patients on maintenance dialysis, Psychology, Health & Medicine, 1-9, iFirst Article.

Thompson, P. D., D. Buchner, *et al.,* (2003). Exercise and physical activity in the prevention and treatment of atherosclerotic cardiovascular disease: a statement from the Council on Clinical Cardiology (Subcommittee on Exercise, Rehabilitation, and Prevention) and the Council on Nutrition, Physical Activity, and Metabolism (Subcommittee on Physical Activity). Circulation 107(24): 3109-3116.

Tsai, Y. C., C. C. Hung, *et al.,* (2010). Quality of life predicts risks of end-stage renal disease and mortality in patients with chronic kidney disease. Nephrology Dialysis Transplantation 25(5): 1621-1626.

Ugurlu, N., D. Bastug, *et al.,* (2012). Determining quality of life, depression and anxiety levels of hemodialysis patients. HealthMed 6(8): 2860-2869.

Unruh, M., R. Benz, *et al.,* (2004). Effects of hemodialysis dose and membrane flux on health-related quality of life in the HEMO Study. Kidney International 66(1): 355-366.

Unruh, M. L. and R. Hess (2007). Assessment of health-related quality of life among patients with chronic kidney disease. Adv Chronic Kidney Dis 14(4): 345-352.

Van Manen, J. G., J. C. Korevaar, *et al.,* (2003). Adjustment for comorbidity in studies on health status in ESRD patients: which comorbidity index to use? Journal of the American Society of Nephrology 14(2): 478-485.

Ware, J. E., Jr. and C. D. Sherbourne (1992). The MOS 36-item short-form health survey (SF-36). I. Conceptual framework and item selection. Med Care 30(6): 473-483.

Ware, J. E., W. H. Rogers, *et al.,* (1986). Comparison of Health Outcomes at a Health Maintenance Organization with Those of Fee-for-Service Care. Lancet 1(8488): 1017-1022.

Weiner, S., N. G. Kutner, *et al.,* (2010). Improving psychosocial health in hemodialysis patients after a disaster. Soc Work Health Care 49(6): 513-525.

Wright, J. G. and A. R. Feinstein (1992). A Comparative Contrast of Clinimetric and Psychometric Methods for Constructing Indexes and Rating-Scales. J Clin Epidemiol 45(11): 1201-1218.

Wu, A. W., N. E. Fink, *et al.,* (2001). Developing a health-related quality-of-life measure for end-stage renal disease: The CHOICE Health Experience Questionnaire. Am J Kidney Dis 37(1): 11-21.

Wyld, M., R. L. Morton, *et al.,* (2012). A systematic review and meta-analysis of utility-based quality of life in chronic kidney disease treatments. PLoS Med 9(9): e1001307.

Yen, M., T. C. Lin, *et al.,* (2011). Measuring quality of life in chronic kidney disease patients: reflections and prospects. Hu Li Za Zhi 58(2): 5-9.

CHAPTER 4

Health-Related Quality of Life Outcomes Among Patients on Maintenance Dialysis

Haikel A. Lim and Konstadina Griva[*]

Department of Psychology, National University of Singapore, Singapore

Abstract: More patients with end-stage kidney disease (ESKD) are becoming increasingly dependent on lifelong dialysis as their only means of renal replacement therapy. However, despite the improvements in dialysis techniques/procedures and care, there are still high mortality rates, which are significantly predicted by a lowered quality of life (QoL). This chapter, therefore, addresses QoL issues in ESKD. We first explore the various issues surrounding QoL in dialysis research. We then briefly review the empirical findings and limitations in this area. We end by proposing applications of QoL research in clinical settings, and examine empirical research that might potentially assist patients with decision-making for different treatment modalities.

Keywords: Quality of life, end-stage kidney disease, dialysis, haemodialysis, peritoneal dialysis, treatment modalities, clinical applications.

INTRODUCTION

End-stage kidney disease (ESKD) is a physically and psychosocially debilitating chronic illness that involves the irreversible loss of kidney function. Patients who suffer from ESKD have several electrolyte, metabolic, and endocrine disorders that can only be mitigated with dialysis or renal transplantation (Axelsson, Randers, Jacobson, & Klang, 2012). For those unable to have a transplant, or whose transplants fail to take, dialysis is a lifelong treatment (Billington, Simpson, Unwin, Bray, & Giles, 2008).

Dialysis involves the removal of toxins and excess fluid from the blood, either *via* the use of a machine (haemodialysis; HD), or *via* the body's abdominal cavity as a

*Address correspondence to Konstadina Griva: Faculty of Arts & Social Sciences, Department of Psychology, National University of Singapore, Singapore; Tel: +65 65163156; Fax: +65 6773-1843; E-mail: psygk@nus.edu.sg

natural filter (peritoneal dialysis; PD). The dialysis regimen is relentless and complex: it involves invasive and painful procedures, alongside strict fluid and diet restrictions, and the management of multiple medications (Hailey & Moss, 2000). Poor adherence is therefore common in dialysis (Leggat *et al.*, 1998) and is coupled with dire consequences such as lowered survival and increased hospitalization (Saran *et al.*, 2003). Thus, mortality rates remain high in this population, despite continuing improvements in dialysis techniques/procedures and care. While a majority of these cases are due to cardiovascular complications, many patients also opt to abate dialysis (Davison, & Jhangri, 2005), citing an increasing burden of dialysis and a deteriorating quality of life (QoL; Ashby *et al.*, 2005).

This chapter is divided into three sections. In the first section, we present the various issues involved in QoL research on dialysis patients. In the second section, we briefly review the empirical findings and limitations in the specific area. In the final section of this chapter, we propose applications of QoL research in clinical settings and examine empirical research that can assist patients with decision-making for different treatment modalities.

THE IMPORTANCE OF QUALITY OF LIFE

Patient-reported outcomes such as QoL are important markers to evaluate effectiveness of ESKD treatment (Bakewell, Higgins, & Edmunds, 2002). Their importance is underlined by strong associations between poor QoL and clinical endpoints (Afsar, Elsurer, Sezer, & Ozdemir, 2009; Birmelé, Le Gall, Sautenet, Aguerre, & Camus, 2012; Santos, Daher, Silva, Libório, & Kerr, 2009). Several large dialysis cohort studies have shown that QoL scores are strong predictors of hospitalisation and mortality (Kalantar-Zadeh, Kopple, Block, & Humphreys, 2001; Lowrie, Curtin, LePain, & Schatell, 2003; Mapes *et al.*, 2004). For instance, in a prospective study of 1000 HD patients, a five-point decrease in the SF-36 physical component summary (PCS) scores resulted in a 5.8% increase in the hospitalisation rate and a 10% increase in death risk, and a similar decrease in the mental component summary (MCS) scores correlated with a 2% increase in hospitalisation rates (DeOreo, 1997). Further, in a large prospective study of 17,236 HD patients in the United States, Europe, and Japan, five-point increase in the PCS, MCS, and kidney disease-specific subscale scores of the KDQoL-SF were associated with a 4–8% reduction in risk of hospitalisation, and a 9–29% reduction in mortality (Mapes *et al.*, 2004).

There is also a growing recognition that maintaining QoL may become particularly important in patient segments that are unlikely to receive a renal transplant such as elderly patients, and who will live on dialysis until their end of life. In fact, dialysis patients, irrespective of age, are willing to trade less living time for better quality of life (Jhamb *et al.*, 2011; Tsevat *et al.*, 1998); nephrologists, therefore, place more weight on quality of life than mortality and morbidity in recommending dialysis modalities (Mendelssohn, Mullaney, Jung, Blake, & Mehta, 2001). Various efforts have thus been initiated to improve patients' quality of life, such as adjusting dialysis prescription, controlling comorbidities, treating anemia and alleviating depression (Ross, Hollen, & Fitzgerald, 2006).

Issues Surrounding Quality of Life in Dialysis

As indicated elsewhere in this book (see Chapter 2), QoL is a difficult concept to define. One of the most widely-used definitions of QoL in research (Berlim *et al.*, 2006) is proposed by the World Health Organization (WHO): 'the individual's perception of his or her position in life, taking into account culturally-specific contexts and value systems, and his goals, expectations, parameters, and social relations' (Harper, & Power, 1998). However, in a clinical setting, QoL is often defined in relation to health and disease, and is typically referred to as health-related quality of life (HRQoL). QoL, therefore, seems to broadly refer to subjective assessments of an individual's well-being that involve both health and non-health related dimensions. However, despite the increasing use of QoL outcomes in research and clinical practice, no consensus exists concerning the definition or the measurements of this multidimensional construct, with only a very small proportion examining the conceptual and operational definitions (Cagney *et al.*, 2000).

This lack of a consensus has led to researchers using different definitions, and hence differing measures, of QoL to suit their research question (see Dean, 1990 for a further explication). When logistically possible, a combined approach, integrating generic QoL scales with disease-specific ones, is recommended (Saban *et al.*, 2008). However, most research done on an ESKD population focuses either on generic or disease-specific QoL.

Some researchers adopt a more encompassing global definition of QoL, employing the use of generic instruments that measure either overall QoL, *e.g.,* the Satisfaction with Life Scale (SWLS; Diener, Emmons, Larsen, & Griffin, 1985) and the WHO Quality of Life Scale 26-item Short Version (WHOQoL-BREF; Harper, & Power, 1998); general health related QoL, *e.g.,* the Medical Outcomes Scale (SF-36; Ware, Jr. & Sherbourne, 1992); or mental health QoL, *e.g.,* the Beck Depression Inventory (BDI; Beck, Ward, & Mendelson, 1961). These measures are broadly applicable across different patient populations, types and severity of diseases/conditions and/ or medical treatments (Patrick, & Deyo, 1989). They allow for comparisons across patient groups (Guyatt, & Jaeschke, 1990), but fail to focus adequately on the particular problems or issues more pertinent for the patient population in question (Tsevat *et al.*, 1994). They may also not be sensitive enough, or appropriately targeted, to detect small yet clinically important changes.

Other researchers focus on disease-specific HRQoL, which tend to be more sensitive to issues or concerns more specific to patients undergoing dialysis group than generic instruments, but do not allow comparisons across different patient groups (Guyatt, Veldhuyzen Van Zanten, Feeny, & Patrick, 1989). Examples of these include the Kidney Disease Quality-of-Life Instrument (KDQoL; Hays, Kallich, Mapes, Coons, & Carter, 1994) and the Kidney Disease Questionnaire (KDQ; Laupacis, Muirhead, Kcown, & Wong, 1992). All the aforementioned instruments represent the more frequently used measures assessing QoL in patients with ESKD (see Bowling, 2001; Cagney *et al.*, 2000; Chan *et al.*, 2012; Edgell *et al.*, 1996, for detailed reviews). For a further explication on the various instruments, we suggest referring to Chapter 3 of this book.

EMPIRICAL FINDINGS IN QUALITY OF LIFE RESEARCH ON DIALYSIS

This section highlights the factors shown to be associated with QoL in dialysis population. Most of the research on QoL outcomes has been based on only on adult patients that represent the majority of ESKD patients, with only handful of studies on paediatric or adolescent patients on dialysis (Gerson *et al.*, 2006; Goldstein, Gerson, Goldman, & Furth, 2006). Thus, in our selective overview, we highlight studies on adult patients and exclude evidence from paediatric patients (for information, see Gerson *et al.*, 2004; Roumelioti *et al.*, 2010). We will also leave out studies that focus on depression (which overlap with the mental dimension of QoL) as these are the foci of other systematic reviews (Chan, Steel, *et al.*, 2011a; see Lew & Piraino, 2005).

Factors associated with QoL in dialysis

Research has identified several factors that are associated with QoL in dialysis patients. These include socio-demographic, clinical and psychosocial factors.

Socio-Demographic Factors

Several studies have shown that socio-demographic factors such as age, gender, ethnicity, socioeconomic status (SES), relationship status, and employment are associated with HRQoL. In general, physical HRQoL seems to deteriorate with age, as seen in most studies on dialysis patients (Mingardi *et al.*, 1999; Moreno, López-Gómez, Sanz-Guajardo, Jofré, & Valderrábano, 1996). However, research has also shown that emotional QoL may be elevated in elderly dialysis patients (Afsar, Elsurer, Sezer, *et al.*, 2009; Evans *et al.*, 1985; Ifudu, Dawood, Homel, & Friedman, 1996; Singer, Martin, & Kelner, 1999; Álvares, Cesar, Acurcio, Andrade, & Cherchiglia, 2012). Differences in health expectations and the ability to accept and adapt to worsening health status/increasing infirmity may explain the QoL differences between older and younger dialysis patients. Older patients may show greater resilience to deteriorating health as this is seen as a normal and expected consequence of aging.

Research on ethnicity and QoL has been somewhat more inconclusive. Studies have shown that African Americans on HD report better heath status and quality of life on selected measures as compared to Caucasians (Hicks, Cleary, Epstein, & Ayanian, 2004), Hispanics, and Asians (Unruh *et al.*, 2004). In contrast, Kutner, Zhang, and Brogan (2005) found that African American patients on HD did not report higher perceived quality of life than their Caucasian counterparts. In another study, Bakewell, Higgins, and Edmunds (2002) found that white Europeans on dialysis report better outcomes in physical health, mental health, and kidney disease specific issues as compared to Asians.

In HD patients, studies have consistently shown that lower SES and lower education levels are correlated with lower SF-36 scores (Caskey *et al.*, 2003; Kao *et al.*, 2009; Moreno *et al.*, 1996; Sesso, Rodrigues-Neto, & Ferraz, 2003; Álvares *et al.*, 2012). Studies have also consistently shown that employed HD patients reported better functioning and HRQoL as compared to dialysis patients that were not (Curtin, Oberley, Sacksteder, & Friedman, 1996; Holley & Nespor, 1994; Porter *et al.*, 2012).

It is also interesting to note that female ESKD patients generally show lowered levels of HRQoL (Mingardi *et al.*, 1999; Sathvik, Parthasarathi, Narahari, & Gurudev, 2008; Valderrábano, Jofré, & López-Gómez, 2001). In one study, HD patients who were married were also likely to report better outcomes in HRQoL as compared to patients who were not married (Mingardi *et al.*, 1999), while other studies have found no effect of marriage (Lopes *et al.*, 2007; Merkus *et al.*, 1997).

Clinical Factors

Research on HD patients has identified clinical and biochemical markers associated with HRQoL, primarily for the physical QoL dimensions. Haemoglobin, a marker of anemia that typically accompanies ESKD, is strongly associated with physical functioning and wellbeing (Mujais *et al.*, 2009; Plantinga *et al.*, 2007). Increasing haemoglobin levels through medication and erythropoietin treatment have been shown to produce concomitant improvements in reported levels of energy and stamina, and higher life participation (Chan, Brooks, *et al.*, 2011; Hansen, Chin, Blalock, & Joy, 2009).

Nutritional biomarkers like albumin, normalized protein catabolic rate (a measure of protein nutrition), and body mass index are most closely associated with physical SF-36 PCS scores (Kalantar-Zadeh *et al.*, 2001; Ohri-Vachaspati & Sehgal, 1999; Spiegel, Melmed, Robbins, & Esrailian, 2008). Inadequate protein nutrition has also been associated with poor physical functioning KDQoL scores (Ohri-Vachaspati, & Sehgal, 1999). Further, other research has shown that lowered SF-36 scores are correlated with lowered self-reported appetite scores (Zabel, Ash, King, Juffs, & Bauer, 2012).

Interventions structured around nutrition and dietary support have also yielded significant improvement in QoL scores (Campbell, Ash, & Bauer, 2008). In contrast, mineral metabolism indices such as calcium-phosphorous product (a measure of adherence to diet and medication) and parathyroid hormone levels (a measure of calcium levels in the blood) were found to be poorly associated with the HRQoL (Mingardi *et al.*, 1999).

Studies that have examined the relationship between dialysis adequacy and HRQoL measures have produced mixed findings. Some studies report associations with generic health QoL (Cleary & Drennan, 2005; Morsch, Gonçalves, & Barros, 2006) and kidney disease-specific QoL scales (Korevaar *et al.*, 2002), while others failing to find significant associations (Lopes *et al.*, 2007; Mingardi *et al.*, 1999; Wang *et al.*, 2008).

The variable most consistently associated with QoL is comorbid burden and multi-morbidity. Increased number of comorbidities (*e.g.*, cardiovascular diseases, peropheral vascular diseases, hypertension and diabetes), understandably, adversely affects physical QoL (Diaz-Buxo, Lowrie, Lew, Zhang, & Lazarus, 2000; Stojanovic, Ilic, & Stefanovic, 2006) and may also deduct from emotional QoL (Fortin *et al.*, 2004).

A brief note should also be made on other medical factors more closely related to organizational health care structures, rather than disease, that have recently been highlighted as potential QoL determinants. For example, the time taken to travel to dialysis centres is associated with HD patients' lowered QoL and impaired clinical outcomes (Diamant *et al.,* 2010; Moist *et al.,* 2008). Also, early and planned referral to dialysis has been shown to be associated with better QoL outcomes (Caskey *et al.*, 2003; Loos, Briançon, Frimat, Hanesse, & Kessler, 2003; White, Pilkey, Lam, & Holland, 2002). Pre-dialysis care allows patients to prepare for dialysis initiation and undergo access procedures in time which may in turn facilitate the transition to life on dialysis and thus favourable QoL outcomes. When patients are diagnosed late and/or when dialysis onset is more precipitous, *e.g.,* emergency dialysis using temporary access, the effects on QoL are more pronounced.

Psychosocial Factors

The ESKD literature has suggested that psychological factors are associated with HRQoL in HD patients: specifically, depression, perception of illness effects and social support have been linked to QoL and mortality in dialysis patients (Kimmel, 2000). In addition, anxiety disorders have also been found to be associated with lower levels of QoL (Cukor *et al.*, 2008). A study by Kimmel, Thamer, Richard, and Ray (1998) found that rate of mood disorders in patients on HD is substantially higher as compared to other chronic medical conditions.

There is substantial variation in the estimated prevalence of depression (meeting the diagnostic criteria for mood disorder) in HD patients, which is estimated to range from 12-40% depending on the criteria used (Hinrichsen, Lieberman, Pollack, & Steinberg, 1989). The observed wide range in the estimate of depression is due to the difficulties in assessing and diagnosing depression in ESKD. Assessment and diagnosis of depression in dialysis patients are problematic because of the similarities between the somatic symptoms of depression and physical symptoms of renal failure and side effects of renal replacement therapy (Kimmel, 2000), studies have consistently shown that depression has been linked to diminished HRQoL and an increase in mortality rates in ESKD patient (Kimmel, Weihs, & Peterson, 1993; Martin & Thompson, 2000; Peterson *et al.*, 1991), while others have not shown such an association (Christensen, Wiebe, Smith, & Turner, 1994).

In contrast to depression, anxiety disorders have received little attention in the ESKD population despite the estimated prevalence of anxiety disorders at 30% in the HD population (Taskapan *et al.*, 2005). Research has shown that anxiety disorders have a negative effect on QoL of patients with physical illnesses such as hypertension, cardiac disease, thyroid disease, and diabetes (Sareen *et al.*, 2006). However, the specific effects of anxiety disorders on HRQoL of ESKD patients have not been well documented (Cukor, Cohen, Peterson, & Kimmel, 2007). Only two studies found that HD patients with pure anxiety disorders (*i.e.,* no other comorbid psychiatric disorders) scored lower on the mean total KDQoL score (*i.e.*, reported lower quality of life) as compared to HD patients with no psychopathology (Cukor *et al.*, 2008, 2007).

Studies have shown that dialysis patients perceiving greater illness intrusiveness of their kidney disease report poorer emotional well-being (Sacks, Peterson, & Kimmel, 1990), poorer satisfaction with life, and poorer functioning (Kimmel *et al.*, 1995). Patient perceptions of illness and treatment are also strongly associated with QoL (Griva, Jayasena, Davenport, Harrison, & Newman, 2009; Timmers *et al.*, 2008). Beliefs about the treatments are likely to be of particular importance in ESKD since dialysis modalities differ significantly in the demands they imposed upon patients. Qualitative investigations have shown that HD is commonly perceived as extremely demanding, burdensome, and disruptive across personal, work, family, and social facets of life. That these beliefs not only dominate patients' experience with ESKD (Gregory, Way, Hutchinson, Barrett, & Parfrey, 1998; Krespi, Bone, Ahmad, Worthington, & Salmon, 2004), but are also associated with QoL outcomes (Griva *et al.*, 2009).

Patients who perceive themselves as having control over their HD have better SEIQoL scores (Tovbin, Gidron, Jean, Granovsky, & Schnieder, 2003). Control perception, such as locus of control (LoC), is related with QoL. Internal LoC has been show to be associated with higher QoL in both PD and HD patients (Birmelé *et al.*, 2012; Pucheu, Consoli, D'Auzac, Français, & Issad, 2004; Theofilou, 2012). Opposite findings of higher QoL with external LoC have also been reported (Billington *et al.*, 2008; Martin & Thompson, 2000).

Patients who perceive themselves as having social support, that is, belonging to a network of affection, mutual aid, and obligation (Kimmel, 2000), have more positive QoL outcomes (Plantinga *et al.*, 2010; Tovbin *et al.*, 2003). Physical support (assistance with dialysis) has also shown to reduce the symptoms and dialysis burden subscales in dialysis patients (Billington *et al.*, 2008). Thus, support and interaction with health care providers are also important in QoL (Beder, 2008; Kliger, & Finkelstein, 2009; Lacson *et al.*, 2009).

Coping is also a particularly salient concept in patient outcomes. ESKD and dialysis is a traumatic experience that brings much stress to the patient, and understandably a lowered QoL. The inability to cope, or the use of maladaptive coping strategies, have been associated with lowered QoL for HD patients (Birmelé et al., 2012). PD patients who employed the use of emotional-focused coping were found to have lowered KDQoL MCS scores; however, neither physical nor mental QoL scores were linked to the use of problem-focused coping (Pucheu et al., 2004). Positive religious coping was associated with better WHOQoL-BREF scores, while religious struggle had inverse correlations to QoL (Ramirez et al., 2012). Coping skills training programs have thus been shown to improve depression and QoL in dialysis patients (Tsay, Lee, & Lee, 2005).

ESKD is typically accompanied by several symptoms; most notably fatigue and lethargy, muscle weakness, generalized itching, loss of appetite, nausea, and vomiting. Symptoms improve, are do not resolved, with the initiation of dialysis. Dialysis treatments are quite intrusive and are typically associated with symptoms such as pain, fatigue and sleep disturbances, these symptoms deduct from QoL and adjustment outcomes (Davison, & Jhangri, 2010; Yarlas et al., 2011). Side effects, such as sexual dysfunction, have similar negative effects on QoL (Afsar, Elsurer, Eyileten, Yilmaz, & Caglar, 2009; Fernandes et al., 2010; Lew-Starowicz, & Gellert, 2009).

This selective overview of literature highlights the importance of a range of socio-demographic, biomedical and psychological variables in determining QoL. However, it is worthwhile to note, at this juncture, that the variables associated with QoL, mentioned above, interact in a myriad of complex combinations and should not be viewed as independent determinants of QoL.

APPLICATIONS OF QUALITY OF LIFE MEASURES IN DIALYSIS

There are a number of ways in which QoL measures can and have been used in research, and this section of the chapter will briefly highlight a few applications.

Quality of Life Measures in Clinical Settings

As QoL improvements have also been associated with reduced costs because of the improved prognosis (Hamel et al., 1997), it is thus important for clinicians to continually track QoL outcomes at different points in patient treatment (Wu et al., 2004). We outline a few reasons below:

Understanding Perceived Symptoms

QoL outcomes are also closely related to other important clinical aspects (Kusztal, Nowak, Magott-Procelewska, Weyde, & Penar, 2003): one study showed that ESKD-related symptoms bothering dialysis patients were negatively related with KDQoL-SF scores but not necessarily clinical variables like serum albumin and haemoglobin (Thong *et al.*, 2009). Depending on the modality, changes in QoL would allow clinicians to ascertain a holistic assessment of the impact of the treatment on the patient's life, specifically patient satisfaction, and burden of disease (Gayle, Soyibo, Gilbert, Manzanares, & Barton, 2009). This would allow for more informed suggestions and decisions on patient care targeted at improving QoL.

Associations with Adherence

Further, while the direction of causality has yet to be determined, QoL outcomes seem to be correlated with adherence (Chiu *et al.*, 2009). For example, non-adherence in HD patients was related to lower SF-36 and higher BDI scores (Akman *et al.*, 2007), and the dialysis staff encouragement subscale of the KDQoL-SF was related to better fluid control adherence (Yokoyama *et al.*, 2009).

Predicting Global Outcomes

As described earlier in this chapter, perhaps the most important reason for the inclusion of QoL outcomes in clinical settings is their prognostic value for clinical outcomes (Afsar, Elsurer, Sezer, *et al.*, 2009; Birmelé *et al.*, 2012; Peng *et al.*, 2010; Santos *et al.*, 2009; Tsai *et al.*, 2010). These highlight the need for regular monitoring of QoL in clinical settings so as to identify early patients with QoL impairment and provide support as needed. This can ultimately feed into better patient management and care (see Dhingra, & Laski, 2003 for further explication).

Guiding Interventions

While there have been no specific interventions targeted at increasing QoL outcomes, most interventions use QoL outcomes as secondary measures to evaluate the effectiveness of interventions. We provide a selective overview of various interventions that have included QoL endpoints.

Improving Clinical Endpoints

Some interventions are targeted primarily at improving mortality, using QoL outcomes as proxies to track progress and effectiveness. For example, a programme done on 918 HD patients, called Right Start, focused on medical needs, patient education and support, has yielded significant benefits in terms of improved SF-36 MCS scores, and lowered mortality and hospitalisation rates (Wingard *et al.*, 2007).

Improving Depression

As depression has come up as a frequent comorbidity in ESKD, interventions using QoL outcomes as proxies have also been developed to look at ways to improve depressive symptoms, treating major depression *via* a cognitive-behavioural group therapy over 9 months intervention lowered BDI and raised KDQoL-SF scores (Duarte, Ciconelli, & Sesso, 2005; Duarte, Miyazaki, Blay, & Sesso, 2009). Further, a symptom targeted intervention (STI) managing depressed mood showed not only lowered BDI scores but also increased SF-36 PCS and MCS scores (Yarlas *et al.*, 2011).

Improving Nutrition

As nutrition has come up as a good predictor of mortality, QoL outcomes have also be used as proxies in interventions targeted at improving nutrition in dialysis patients. One such intervention has shown increased SF-36 PCS (Spiegel *et al.*, 2008) and increased KDQoL scores (Campbell *et al.*, 2008). Another, the group Nutrition Education Program done over 5 months during HD treatment, have shown higher SF-36 scores as compared to controls (Wiser, Shane, McGuigan, Memken, & Olsson, 1997).

Improving Treatment

In addition to being used as indicators for current treatments QoL outcomes can, be used to measure the feasibility of new treatment methods. For example, a trial using human growth hormone treatment showed simultaneous increases in lean body mass, serum albumin levels, and SF-36 PCS scores in HD patients (Feldt-Rasmussen *et al.*, 2007). Also, an intervention targeted at seeking the effectiveness of HD dose and membrane flux showed slight increases in SF-36 PCS scores but no clinically significant change on other QoL outcomes (M. Unruh *et al.*, 2004) improved SF-36 MCS scores have been used to promote certain physical activity interventions like a Tai Chi Wu-style intervention on PD patients (Mustata *et al.*, 2005).

Improving Physical Activity

The bulk of interventions done in dialysis patients using QoL outcomes as secondary measures of efficacy have been focused on improving physical activity, primarily because physical activity seems to improve both QoL and mortality (Cheema, & Singh, 2005). For example, one intervention found that SF-36 PCS scores improved as a result of physical activity counselling and encouragement (Painter, Carlson, Carey, Paul, & Myll, 2000a). Patients with low SF-36 PCS scores benefitted the most from exercise counselling in the Renal Exercise Demonstration Project (Painter, Carlson, Carey, Paul, & Myll, 2000b), but there seemed to be no effect for high-functioning patients (DePaul, Moreland, Eager, & Clase, 2002). In other studies, SF-36 scores increased following a twelve-week (Reboredo *et al.*, 2010) and a year-long intervention (Capitanini *et al.*, 2008), which is cross-culturally supported (Jang & Kim, 2009).

In addition to SF-36 score improvements that denote intervention effectiveness, a six-week physical lifestyle rehabilitation program (The Life Readiness Program) showed improved KDQoL-SF physical function scores (Tawney *et al.*, 2000) in HD; however, another intervention showed that physical exercise alone showed no difference on KDQoL-SF (Parsons, Toffelmire, & King-VanVlack, 2006), although this might have been the result of not controlling for confounds (Hsieh & Lee, 2007). Physical exercise interventions have also improved KDQoL in CAPD patients (Lo *et al.*, 1998).

Improving Management

QoL outcomes can also be used as secondary measures in interventions targeted at improving treatment adherence: a group-based intervention targeting negative illness perceptions, improving self-care behaviours, and improving patient education showed lowered BDI and improved SF-36 scores (Lii, Tsay, & Wang, 2007). A nurse-led case management programme was applied effectively to PD patients and found to enhance wellbeing and KDQoL-SF scores in the transition from hospital to home (Chow, & Wong, 2010). While few studies have used the aforementioned QoL measures, we foresee that with the integration of QoL outcomes in clinical settings, more research and trials will target such psychosocial factors (*e.g.*, Griva *et al.*, 2011).

Decision-Making for Treatment Modalities

Undeniably, the greatest impact for QoL as an outcome measure is in the field of decision-making for treatment (Ahmed, *et al.*, 1999). ESKD patients may face multiple treatment-related decisions on the course of kidney disease; for instance decisions on whether to start on dialysis, which dialysis modality to opt for, or whether or not pursue transplantation. In the absence of medical contra-indications, these decisions become a matter of personal choice. Such a decision requires thoughtful consideration of the value a patient, and potentially their family, places on the potential gains or losses in QoL associated with each treatment.

Moreover, considerations related to QoL are also important for other parties that may be involved in decision making process, *i.e.,* families, partners, health care professionals. QoL considerations can inform recommendations made to patients or the decisions caregivers may be making on behalf of the patients, as in the case of pediatric patients (Greenhalgh, Long, & Flynn, 2005). QoL outcome measures may also help to bring more novel treatment alternatives into the foray (Williams *et al.*, 2004) or at least push for more clinical trials to be done on their effectiveness.

The final portion of this chapter will, thus, selectively review literature on the differences in QoL between treatment modalities.

Dialysis vs. Healthy Populations

Dialysis undoubtedly places a strain on individuals, and understandably, the observed mean QoL scores of dialysis patients are lower than those in healthy populations (Afsar, Elsurer, Eyileten, *et al.*, 2009; Chan, Brooks, Erlich, Chow, & Suranyi, 2009; Kutner, Zhang, & McClellan, 2000). For example, HD patients have lowered PCS SF-36 scores (Cleary, & Drennan, 2005) and impaired SEIQoL scores (Pugh-Clarke, Naish, & Mercer, 2006) when compared to normal populations. However, KDQoL mental scores are similar both in dialysis and normal geriatric populations (Lamping *et al.*, 2000).

In PD patients, ESKD-specific QoL measures were found to steadily decline during a two-year period, with the most significant changes being general health symptoms/problems, burden of kidney disease, emotional wellbeing, and patient satisfaction (Bakewell *et al.*, 2002). This is contrasted to findings that show "several QoL dimensions were systematically better for PD patients during the follow-up, particularly burden of kidney disease, encouragement from staff, and satisfaction with care" (De Abreu, Walker, Sesso, & Ferraz, 2011). However, research has also found seasonal variability of PCS SF-36 scores in HD patients, which seem to be higher in July compared to January (Afsar, & Kirkpantur, 2012).

Dialysis vs. Transplant Populations

Kidney transplants, if available, are often presented as the best option (Evans *et al.*, 1985; Álvares *et al.*, 2012) because of QoL measures have shown to improve (Landreneau, Lee, & Landreneau, 2010) to that of normal populations after transplant (Maglakelidze, Pantsulaia, Tchokhonelidze, Managadze, & Chkhotua, 2011; Rambod, Shabani, Shokrpour, Rafii, & Mohammadalliha, 2011). WHOQoL-BREF scores are significantly lower for HD (Sathvik *et al.*, 2008) and PD patients as compared to transplant patients (Niu & Li, 2005). This is similar for SF-36 scores, although differences in QoL may be explained by age and the prevalence of diabetes (Liem, Bosch, Arends, Heijenbrok-Kal, & Hunink, 2007). Regardless, KDQoL scores have shown to be higher in transplant, than dialysis patients (Kovacs *et al.*, 2011).

It is perhaps important to note some issues that might have influenced the abovementioned results. There may be issues of cultural specificity, as there seems to be no difference on SF-36 scores between dialysis and transplant patients in a Turkish sample (Sayin, Mutluay, & Sindel, 2007). Further, the success of the transplant graft may also affect QoL (Decker *et al.*, 2008); for example, our past research has shown that QoL decreases in patients with failed transplants (Griva, Davenport, Harrison, & Newman, 2012).

HD vs. PD

With PD generating more traction as a more viable and cost effective method of dialysis, QoL outcomes can also help to patients determine which modality they prefer. However, research on the differences between the two treatment modalities appears split. On one hand, there seem to be no differences in QoL between the groups (Sayin *et al.*, 2007; Tucker, Ziller, Smith, Mars, & Coons, 1991), specifically SF-36 MCS scores ct on HRQo(Bipath, Govender, & Viljoen, 2008; Álvares *et al.*, 2012) and even PCS scores (Bipath *et al.*, 2008). This is true for both generic measures (Liem, Bosch, & Hunink, 2008; Wasserfallen *et al.*, 2004), and disease-specific ones, like the KDQoL-SF (De Abreu *et al.*, 2011).

On the other hand, some have found an increased QoL for PD as compared to HD populations (Mau, Chiu, Chang, Hwang, & Hwang, 2008), with PD patients having higher mental KDQoL scores and slightly lowered mortality and hospitalisation rates (Harris, Lamping, Brown, & Constantinovici, 2002). HD patients have also indicated lower disease-specific QoL as compared to PD patients (Ginieri-Coccossis, Theofilou, Synodinou, Tomaras, & Soldatos, 2008), although the opposite effects have also been found (Fructuoso, Castro, Oliveira, Prata, & Morgado, 2011). Within PD modalities, CCPD (continuous cycling PD) patients score worse for on disease-specific physical functioning QoL measures, but better for mental function, than either CAPD (continuous ambulatory PD) or HD patients (Diaz-Buxo *et al.*, 2000).

Unfortunately, there is still insufficient data to allow conclusions to be drawn about the relative effectiveness of PD as compared with HD for adults (Kutner, 2004; Rabindranath *et al.*, 2006; Vale *et al.*, 2004). A recent review concluded that despite PD patients rating higher QoL, and HD patients enjoying better physical QoL over time, there is no simple answer to which modality is more effective; central to this debate is just a good understanding of the evidence in the field which would facilitate individual decision-making (Boateng, & East, 2011).

CAPD vs. APD

Unfortunately, there is still insufficient data to allow conclusions to be drawn about the relative effectiveness of different PD modalities (Bowman, & Martin, 1999). Although a recent review has shown that APD appears to have better QoL outcomes than CAPD (Rabindranath *et al.*, 2007), supported by research that showed higher BDI scores in CAPD patients as compared to APD and home HD patients (Griva, Davenport, Harrison, & Newman, 2010), recent studies found no such differences between SF-36 total and subscale scores between both APD and CAPD patients (Bilgic *et al.*, 2011; Guney *et al.*, 2010).

Daily Dialysis

Daily dialysis, which is more cost effective in the long run (Mohr *et al.*, 2001), seems to have the greatest improvement in QoL outcomes (Vos, Zilch, & Kooistra, 2001). Patients receiving daily haemodialysis have increased QoL outcomes, less comorbidity and less hospitalization (Rayment & Bonner, 2008), supported by prospective study findings (Williams *et al.*, 2004). General physical and mental functioning scores of the KDQoL also showed a marked improvement in daily dialysis (Vos *et al.*, 2001). However, more empirical evidence (longitudinal studies with control groups) is required before any conclusions can be drawn (Kutner, 2004).

Hospital vs. Home Dialysis

Any treatment that is conducted outside of the hospital setting, and promotes independence has been associated with greater QoL scores (Loos-Ayav *et al.*, 2008; McFarlane, Bayoumi, Pierratos, & Redelmeier, 2003; Su, Lu, Chen, & Wang, 2009); however, the research has been inconclusive. For example, home HD has been shown to have increased SF-36 scores (Ageborg, Allenius, & Cederfjaall, 2005). In addition, nocturnal HD was associated with clinically and statistically significant improvements in KDQoL scores (Van Eps *et al.*, 2010) in selected kidney-specific QoL domains (Culleton *et al.*, 2007). However, a comparison between nocturnal home HD and PD showed similar KDQOL-SF PCS, MCS, and KDI scores, and no differences between BDI scores, although PD patients seemed to experience better social support but lower sexual function (Fong, Bargman, & Chan, 2007). This is supported by another study that found no differences between KDQoL-SF scores between nocturnal HD and conventional HD patients (Manns *et al.*, 2009).

CONCLUDING REMARKS

This chapter has provided a non-exhaustive selective overview of the issues surrounding QoL measurement in dialysis populations. In our first section, we looked at contemporary issues surrounding QoL in research and the importance of QoL in clinical settings. In the second section, we looked at the empirical findings and the correlations of socio-demographic, clinical, and psychosocial factors with QoL outcomes from frequency used measures. In our third and final section, we reviewed the different ways in which QoL outcomes can be applied in clinical practice and how they can be used to guide interventions and assist with decision-making. We conclude this chapter by proposing future directions for research and practice.

Future Directions

As previously mentioned, much of the research has been done only on adult or geriatric populations; none have yet to be done extensively on a paediatric or adolescent population, nor have these population-specific measures been adequately validated (Goldstein *et al.*, 2006). Another population that we feel deserves more attention by both clinicians and researchers is the QoL of families and caregivers.

Chronic diseases influence both the patients' and their families' lives. ESKD can place restrictions on spouses and families' lives and thrust them into new situations for which they may be unprepared, unwilling, or unable to manage. Partners and family members often play a key caregiving role to people with ESKD, particularly in children and patients receiving home-based dialysis. Patients may depend on family support to maintain their complex treatment regimen, including performing dialysis-related tasks at home, such as machine setup and needling, managing medications, or providing transport to attend in-centre dialysis treatments and medical appointments. Caregivers, especially those of patients on PD, experience a "significant burden and adverse effects on their [QoL]" (Belasco, Barbosa, Bettencourt, Diccini, & Sesso, 2006).

Aside from direct assistance, families of ESKD patients also have to come to terms with having a loved one with a life threatening illness, as well as dealing with changes in family dynamics that may lead to tension and conflict, and the financial strain related to direct costs of treatment or loss of productivity. The on-going stress and worry manifest in elevated rates of depression and anxiety, fatigue, social isolation and poor QoL (Celik, Annagur, Yılmaz, Demir, & Kara, 2012; Low, Smith, Burns, & Jones, 2008; Wiedebusch *et al.*, 2010).

QoL may be an elusive and mystifying construct to define; similarly, QoL outcomes are often difficult to interpret. While we advocate that QoL be used in tandem with other clinical measures, we support the assertion that it does not completely substitute for clinical outcomes (Higginson, & Carr, 2001), and, as we should be used and interpreted specifically with regard to its intended purpose. Only in picking the right instrument for the right aspect of QoL will we be better able to understand the complex issues surrounding QoL in dialysis patients.

ACKNOWLEDGEMENT

None Declared.

CONFLICT OF INTEREST

None Declared.

REFERENCES

Afsar, B., Elsurer, R., Eyileten, T., Yilmaz, M. I., & Caglar, K. (2009). Antibody response following hepatitis B vaccination in dialysis patients: does depression and life quality matter? Vaccine, 27, 5865–5869. doi:10.1016/j.vaccine.2009.07.055

Afsar, B., Elsurer, R., Sezer, S., & Ozdemir, N. F. (2009a). Does metabolic syndrome have an impact on the quality of life and mood of hemodialysis patients? Journal of Renal Nutrition, 19, 365–371. doi:10.1053/j.jrn.2009.01.016

Afsar, B., & Kirkpantur, A. (2012). Are there any seasonal changes of cognitive impairment, depression, sleep disorders and quality of life in hemodialysis patients? General Hospital Psychiatry. doi:10.1016/j.genhosppsych.2012.08.007

Ageborg, M., Allenius, B.-L., & Cederfjaall, C. (2005). Quality of life, self-care and sense of coherence in patients on hemodialysis: A comparative study. Hemodialysis International, 9, 86–87. doi:10.1111/j.1492-7535.2005.1121at.x

Ahmed, S., Addicott, C., Qureshi, M., Pendleton, N., Clague, J. E., & Horan, M. A. (1999). Opinions of elderly people on treatment for end-stage renal disease. Gerontology, 45, 156–159. doi:22078

Akman, B., Uyar, M., Afsar, B., Sezer, S., Ozdemir, F. N., & Haberal, M. (2007). Adherence, depression and quality of life in patients on a renal transplantation waiting list. Transplant International, 20, 682–7. doi:10.1111/j.1432-2277.2007.00495.x

Álvares, J., Cesar, C. C., Acurcio, F. D. A., Andrade, E. I. G., & Cherchiglia, M. L. (2012). Quality of life of patients in renal replacement therapy in Brazil: Comparison of treatment modalities. Quality of Life Research, 21, 983–991. doi:10.1007/s11136-011-0013-6

Ashby, M., op't Hoog, C., Kellehear, A., Kerr, P. G., Brooks, D., Nicholls, K., & Forrest, M. (2005). Renal dialysis abatement: Lessons from a social study. Palliative Medicine, 19, 389–396. doi:10.1191/0269216305pm1043oa

Axelsson, L., Randers, I., Jacobson, S. H., & Klang, B. (2012). Living with haemodialysis when nearing end of life. Scandinavian Journal of Caring Sciences, 26, 45–52. doi:10.1111/j.1471-6712.2011.00902.x

Bakewell, A. B., Higgins, R. M., & Edmunds, M. E. (2002). Quality of life in peritoneal dialysis patients: decline over time and association with clinical outcomes. Kidney International, 61, 239–248. doi:10.1046/j.1523-1755.2002.00096.x

Beck, A. T., Ward, C. H., & Mendelson, M. (1961). An inventory for measuring depression. Archives of General Psychiatry, 4, 561–571. doi:10.1001/archpsyc.1961.01710120031004

Beder, J. (2008). Evaluation research on social work interventions: A study on the impact of social worker staffing. Social Work in Health Care, 47, 1–13. doi:10.1080/00981380801970590

Belasco, A., Barbosa, D., Bettencourt, A. R., Diccini, S., & Sesso, R. C. (2006). Quality of life of family caregivers of elderly patients on hemodialysis and peritoneal dialysis. American Journal of Kidney Diseases, 48, 955–963. doi:10.1053/j.ajkd.2006.08.017

Berlim, M. T., Mattevi, B. S., Duarte, A. P. G., Thomé, F. S., Barros, E. J. G., & Fleck, M. P. (2006). Quality of life and depressive symptoms in patients with major depression and end-stage renal disease: A matched-pair study. Journal of Psychosomatic Research, 61, 731–734. doi:10.1016/j.jpsychores.2006.04.011

Bilgic, A., Akman, B., Sezer, S., Arat, Z., Ozelsancak, R., & Ozdemir, N. (2011). Daytime sleepiness and quality of life in peritoneal dialysis patients. Therapeutic Apheresis and Dialysis, 15, 565–571. doi:10.1111/j.1744-9987.2011.00987.x

Billington, E., Simpson, J., Unwin, J., Bray, D., & Giles, D. (2008). Does hope predict adjustment to end-stage renal failure and consequent dialysis? British Journal of Health Psychology, 13, 683–699. doi:10.1348/135910707X248959

Bipath, P., Govender, C., & Viljoen, M. (2008). A comparison of quality of life in haemodialysis and peritoneal dialysis patients. Journal of Psychology in Africa, 18, 625–632. Retrieved from http://hdl.handle.net/2263/14495

Birmelé, B., Le Gall, A., Sautenet, B., Aguerre, C., & Camus, V. (2012). Clinical, sociodemographic, and psychological correlates of health-related quality of life in chronic hemodialysis patients. Psychosomatics, 53, 30–37. doi:10.1016/j.psym.2011.07.002

Boateng, E. A., & East, L. (2011). The impact of dialysis modality on quality of life: A systematic review. Journal of Renal Care, 37, 190–200. doi:10.1111/j.1755-6686.2011.00244.x

Bowling, A. (2001). Health-related quality of life: Conceptual meaning, use and measurement. In A. Bowling (Ed.), Measuring disease: A review of disease-specific quality of life measurement scales. (Second Edi., pp. 1–23). Buckingham, UK: Open University Press.

Bowman, G. S., & Martin, C. R. (1999). Evidence of life quality in CAPD patients and implications for nursing care: A systematic review. Clinical Effectiveness in Nursing, 3, 112–123. doi:10.1016/S1361-9004(99)80014-4

Cagney, K. A., Wu, A. W., Fink, N. E., Jenckes, M. W., Meyer, K. B., Bass, E. B., & Powe, N. R. (2000). Formal literature review of quality-of-life instruments used in end-stage renal disease. American Journal of Kidney Diseases, 36, 327–336. doi:10.1053/ajkd.2000.8982

Campbell, K. L., Ash, S., & Bauer, J. D. (2008). The impact of nutrition intervention on quality of life in pre-dialysis chronic kidney disease patients. Clinical Nutrition, 27, 537–544. doi:10.1016/j.clnu.2008.05.002

Capitanini, A., Cupisti, A., Mochi, N., Rossini, D., Lupi, A., Michelotti, G., & Rossi, A. (2008). Effects of exercise training on exercise aerobic capacity and quality of life in hemodialysis patients. Journal of Nephrology, 21, 738–743. Retrieved from http://www.ncbi.nlm.nih.gov/pubmed/18949729

Caskey, F. J., Wordsworth, S., Ben, T., De Charro, F. T., Delcroix, C., Dobronravov, V., Van Hamersvelt, H., *et al.* (2003). Early referral and planned initiation of dialysis: What impact on quality of life? Nephrology, Dialysis, Transplantation, 18, 1330–1338. doi:10.1093/ndt/gfg156

Celik, G., Annagur, B. B., Yılmaz, M., Demir, T., & Kara, F. (2012). Are sleep and life quality of family caregivers affected as much as those of hemodialysis patients? General Hospital Psychiatry, 34, 518–524. doi:10.1016/j.genhosppsych.2012.01.013

Chan, R., Brooks, R., Erlich, J., Chow, J., & Suranyi, M. (2009). The effects of kidney-disease-related loss on long-term dialysis patients' depression and quality of life: Positive affect as a mediator. Clinical Journal of the American Society of Nephrology, 4, 160–167. doi:10.2215/CJN.01520308

Chan, R., Brooks, R., Erlich, J., Gallagher, M., Snelling, P., Chow, J., & Suranyi, M. (2011). Studying psychosocial adaptation to end-stage renal disease: The proximal-distal model of health-related outcomes as a base model. Journal of Psychosomatic Research, 70, 455–464. doi:10.1016/j.jpsychores.2010.11.005

Chan, R., Brooks, R., Steel, Z., Heung, T., Erlich, J., Chow, J., & Suranyi, M. (2012). The psychosocial correlates of quality of life in the dialysis population: A systematic review and meta-regression analysis. Quality of Life Research, 21, 563–580. doi:10.1007/s11136-011-9973-9

Chan, R., Steel, Z., Brooks, R., Heung, T., Erlich, J., Chow, J., & Suranyi, M. (2011a). Psychosocial risk and protective factors for depression in the dialysis population: A systematic review and meta-regression analysis. Journal of Psychosomatic Research, 71, 300–310. doi:10.1016/j.jpsychores.2011.05.002

Cheema, B. S. B., & Singh, M. A. F. (2005). Exercise training in patients receiving maintenance hemodialysis: A systematic review of clinical trials. American Journal of Nephrology, 25, 1219–1229. doi:10.1159/000087184

Chiu, Y.-W., Teitelbaum, I., Misra, M., De Leon, E. M., Adzize, T., & Mehrotra, R. (2009). Pill burden, adherence, hyperphosphatemia, and quality of life in maintenance dialysis patients. Clinical Journal of the American Society of Nephrology, 4, 1089–96. doi:10.2215/CJN.00290109

Chow, S. K. Y., & Wong, F. K. Y. (2010). Health-related quality of life in patients undergoing peritoneal dialysis: Effects of a nurse-led case management programme. Journal of Advanced Nursing, 66, 1780–92. doi:10.1111/j.1365-2648.2010.05324.x

Christensen, A. J., Wiebe, J. S., Smith, T. W., & Turner, C. W. (1994). Predictors of survival among hemodialysis patients: Effect of perceived family support. Health Psychology, 13, 521–525. doi:10.1037/0278-6133.13.6.521

Cleary, J., & Drennan, J. (2005). Quality of life of patients on haemodialysis for end-stage renal disease. Journal of Advanced Nursing, 51, 577–586. doi:10.1111/j.1365-2648.2005.03547.x

Cukor, D., Cohen, S. D., Peterson, R. A., & Kimmel, P. L. (2007). Psychosocial aspects of chronic disease: ESRD as a paradigmatic illness. Journal of the American Society of Nephrology, 18, 3042–3055. doi:10.1681/ASN.2007030345

Cukor, D., Coplan, J., Brown, C., Friedman, S., Newville, H., Safier, M., Spielman, L. a, *et al.* (2008). Anxiety disorders in adults treated by hemodialysis: A single-center study. American Journal of Kidney Diseases, 52, 128–136. doi:10.1053/j.ajkd.2008.02.300

Culleton, B. F., Walsh, M. W., Klarenbach, S. W., Mortis, G., Scott-Douglas, N., Quinn, R. R., Tonelli, M., *et al.* (2007). Effect of frequent nocturnal hemodialysis *vs.* conventional hemodialysis on left ventricular mass and quality of life: A randomized controlled trial. Journal of the American Medical Association, 298, 1291–1299. doi:10.1001/jama.298.11.1291

Curtin, R. B., Oberley, E. T., Sacksteder, P., & Friedman, A. (1996). Differences between employed and nonemployed dialysis patients. American Journal of Kidney Diseases, 27, 533–540. doi:10.1016/S0272-6386(96)90164-X

Davison, S. N., & Jhangri, G. S. (2005). The impact of chronic pain on depression, sleep, and the desire to withdraw from dialysis in hemodialysis patients. Journal of Pain and Symptom Management, 30, 465–473. doi:10.1016/j.jpainsymman.2005.05.013

Davison, S. N., & Jhangri, G. S. (2010). Impact of pain and symptom burden on the health-related quality of life of hemodialysis patients. Journal of Pain and Symptom Management, 39, 477–485. doi:10.1016/j.jpainsymman.2009.08.008

De Abreu, M. M., Walker, D. R., Sesso, R. C., & Ferraz, M. B. (2011). Health-related quality of life of patients recieving hemodialysis and peritoneal dialysis in São Paulo, Brazil: a longitudinal study. Value in Health, 14, S119–21. doi:10.1016/j.jval.2011.05.016

Dean, H. E. (1990). Political and ethical implications of using quality of life as an outcome measure. Seminars in Oncology Nursing, 6, 303–308. doi:10.1016/0749-2081(90)90034-3

Decker, O., Overbeck, I., Mohs, A., Bartels, M., Geisse, B., Hauss, J., & Fangmann, J. (2008). Comparison of quality of life of dialysis patients on the waiting list and patients after kidney transplantation. Zeitschrift fur Medizinische Psychologie, 17, 27–30.

DeOreo, P. B. (1997). Hemodialysis patient-assessed functional health status predicts continued survival, hospitalization, and dialysis-attendance compliance. American Journal of Kidney Diseases, 30, 204–212. doi:10.1016/S0272-6386(97)90053-6

DePaul, V., Moreland, J., Eager, T., & Clase, C. M. (2002). The effectiveness of aerobic and muscle strength training in patients receiving hemodialysis and EPO: A randomized controlled trial. American Journal of Kidney Diseases, 40, 1219–1229. doi:10.1053/ajkd.2002.36887

Dhingra, H., & Laski, M. E. (2003). Outcomes research in dialysis. Seminars in Nephrology, 23, 295–305. doi:10.1016/S0270-9295(03)00065-2

Diamant, M. J., Harwood, L., Movva, S., Wilson, B., Stitt, L., Lindsay, R. M., & Moist, L. M. (2010). A comparison of quality of life and travel-related factors between in-center and satellite-based hemodialysis patients. Clinical Journal of the American Society of Nephrology, 5, 268–274. doi:10.2215/CJN.05190709

Diaz-Buxo, J. A., Lowrie, E. G., Lew, N. L., Zhang, H., & Lazarus, J. M. (2000). Quality-of-life evaluation using Short Form 36: comparison in hemodialysis and peritoneal dialysis patients. American Journal of Kidney Diseases, 35, 293–300. Retrieved from http://www.ncbi.nlm.nih.gov/pubmed/10676729

Diener, E., Emmons, R. A., Larsen, R. J., & Griffin, S. (1985). The satisfaction with life scale. Journal of Personality Assessment, 49, 71–75. doi:10.1207/s15327752jpa4901_13

Duarte, P. S., Ciconelli, R. M., & Sesso, R. C. (2005). Cultural adaptation and validation of the "Kidney Disease and Quality of Life - Short Form (KDQOL-SF^{TM} 1.3)" in Brazil. Brazilian Journal of Medical and Biological Research, 38, 261–270. doi:10.1590/S0100-879X2005000200015

Duarte, P. S., Miyazaki, M. C., Blay, S. L., & Sesso, R. C. (2009). Cognitive-behavioral group therapy is an effective treatment for major depression in hemodialysis patients. Kidney International, 76, 414–421. doi:10.1038/ki.2009.156

Edgell, E. T., Coons, S. J., Carter, W. B., Kallich, J. D., Mapes, D. L., Damush, T. M., & Hays, R. D. (1996). A review of health-related quality-of-life measures used in end-stage renal disease. Clinical Therapeutics, 18, 887–938. doi:10.1016/S0149-2918(96)80049-X

Evans, R. W., Manninen, D. L., Garrison, L. P., Hart, L. G., Blagg, C. R., Gutman, R. A., Hull, A. R., *et al.* (1985). The quality of life of patients with end-stage renal disease. The New England Journal of Medicine, 312, 553–559. doi:10.1056/NEJM198502283120905

Feldt-Rasmussen, B., Lange, M., Sulowicz, W., Gafter, U., Lai, K. N., Wiedemann, J., Christiansen, J. S., *et al.* (2007). Growth hormone treatment during hemodialysis in a randomized trial improves nutrition, quality of life, and cardiovascular risk. Journal of the American Society of Nephrology, 18, 2161–2171. doi:10.1681/ASN.2006111207

Fernandes, G. V., Dos Santos, R. R., Soares, W., De Lima, L. G., De Macêdo, B. S., Da Fonte, J. E., De Carvalho, B. S. P., *et al.* (2010). The impact of erectile dysfunction on the quality of life of men undergoing hemodialysis and its association with depression. The Journal of Sexual Medicine, 7, 4003–4010. doi:10.1111/j.1743-6109.2010.01993.x

Fong, E., Bargman, J. M., & Chan, C. T. (2007). Cross-sectional comparison of quality of life and illness intrusiveness in patients who are treated with nocturnal home hemodialysis *vs.* peritoneal dialysis. Clinical Journal of the American Society of Nephrology, 2, 1195–1200. doi:10.2215/CJN.02260507

Fortin, M., Lapointe, L., Hudon, C., Vanasse, A., Ntetu, A. L., & Maltais, D. (2004). Multimorbidity and quality of life in primary care: A systematic review. Health and Quality of Life Outcomes, 2, 51. doi:10.1186/1477-7525-2-51

Fructuoso, M. R., Castro, R., Oliveira, L., Prata, C., & Morgado, T. (2011). Quality of life in chronic kidney disease. Nefrología, 31, 91–96. doi:10.3265/Nefrologia.pre2010.Jul.10483

Gayle, F., Soyibo, A. K., Gilbert, D. T., Manzanares, J., & Barton, E. N. (2009). Quality of life in end stage renal disease: A multicentre comparative study. The West Indian Medical Journal, 58, 235–242. Retrieved from http://www.ncbi.nlm.nih.gov/pubmed/20043531

Gerson, A. C., Butler, R., Moxey-Mims, M., Wentz, A., Shinnar, S., Lande, M. B., Mendley, S. R., *et al.* (2006). Neurocognitive outcomes in children with chronic kidney disease: Current findings and contemporary endeavors. Mental Retardation and Developmental Disabilities Research Reviews, 12, 208–215. doi:10.1002/mrdd.20116

Gerson, A. C., Hwang, W., Fiorenza, J., Barth, K., Kaskel, F., Weiss, L., Zelikovsky, N., *et al.* (2004). Anemia and health-related quality of life in adolescents with chronic kidney disease. American Journal of Kidney Diseases, 44, 1017–1023. doi:10.1053/j.ajkd.2004.08.024

Ginieri-Coccossis, M., Theofilou, P., Synodinou, C., Tomaras, V., & Soldatos, C. (2008). Quality of life, mental health and health beliefs in haemodialysis and peritoneal dialysis patients: investigating differences in early and later years of current treatment. BMC Nephrology, 9. doi:10.1186/1471-2369-9-14

Goldstein, S. L., Gerson, A. C., Goldman, C. W., & Furth, S. L. (2006). Quality of life for children with chronic kidney disease. Seminars in Nephrology, 26, 114–117. doi:10.1016/j.semnephrol.2005.09.004

Greenhalgh, J., Long, A. F., & Flynn, R. (2005). The use of patient reported outcome measures in routine clinical practice: Lack of impact or lack of theory? Social Science & Medicine, 60, 833–843. doi:10.1016/j.socscimed.2004.06.022

Gregory, D. M., Way, C. Y., Hutchinson, T. A., Barrett, B. J., & Parfrey, P. S. (1998). Patients' perceptions of their experiences with ESRD and hemodialysis treatment. Qualitative Health Research, 8, 764–783. doi:10.1177/104973239800800604

Griva, K., Davenport, A., Harrison, M., & Newman, S. P. (2010). An evaluation of illness, treatment perceptions, and depression in hospital- *vs.* home-based dialysis modalities. Journal of Psychosomatic Research, 69, 363–370. doi:10.1016/j.jpsychores.2010.04.008

Griva, K., Davenport, A., Harrison, M., & Newman, S. P. (2012). The impact of treatment transitions between dialysis and transplantation on illness cognitions and quality of life - A prospective study. British Journal of Health Psychology, 17, 812–827. doi:10.1111/j.2044-8287.2012.02076.x

Griva, K., Jayasena, D., Davenport, A., Harrison, M., & Newman, S. P. (2009). Illness and treatment cognitions and health related quality of life in end stage renal disease. British Journal of Health Psychology, 14, 17–34. doi:10.1348/135910708X292355

Griva, K., Mooppil, N., Seet, P., Krishnan, D. S. P., James, H., & Newman, S. P. (2011). The NKF-NUS hemodialysis trial protocol - a randomized controlled trial to determine the effectiveness of a self management intervention for hemodialysis patients. BMC Nephrology, 12, 4. doi:10.1186/1471-2369-12-4

Guney, I., Solak, Y., Atalay, H., Yazici, R., Altintepe, L., Kara, F., Yeksan, M., *et al.* (2010). Comparison of effects of automated peritoneal dialysis and continuous ambulatory peritoneal dialysis on health-related quality of life, sleep quality, and depression. Hemodialysis International, 14, 515–522. doi:10.1111/j.1542-4758.2010.00465.x

Guyatt, G. H., & Jaeschke, R. (1990). Measurements in clinical trials: Choosing the appropriate approach. Quality of life: Assessments in clinical trials (pp. 37–46). New York, NY, USA: Raven.

Guyatt, G. H., Veldhuyzen Van Zanten, S. J. O., Feeny, D. H., & Patrick, D. L. (1989). Measuring quality of life in clinical trials: A taxonomy and review. Canadian Medical Association Journal, 140, 1441–1448. Retrieved from http://www.pubmedcentral.nih.gov/articlerender.fcgi?artid=1269981&tool=pmcentrez&rendertype=abstract

Hailey, B. J., & Moss, S. B. (2000). Compliance behaviour in patients undergoing haemodialysis: A review of the literature. Psychology, Health & Medicine, 5, 395–406. doi:10.1080/713690222

Hamel, M. B., Phillips, R. S., Davis, R. B., Desbiens, N., Connors, A. F., Teno, J. M., Wenger, N., *et al.* (1997). Outcomes and cost-effectiveness of initiating dialysis and continuing aggressive care in seriously ill hospitalized adults. Annals of Internal Medicine, 127, 195–202. doi: 10.7326/0003-4819-127-3-199708010-00003

Hansen, R. A., Chin, H., Blalock, S., & Joy, M. S. (2009). Predialysis chronic kidney disease: Evaluation of quality of life in clinic patients receiving comprehensive anemia care. Research in Social & Administrative Pharmacy, 5, 143–153. doi:10.1016/j.sapharm.2008.06.004

Harper, A., & Power, M. (1998). Development of the World Health Organisation WHOQOL-BREF quality of life assessment. Psychological Medicine, 28, 551–558.

Harris, S. A. C., Lamping, D. L., Brown, E. A., & Constantinovici, N. (2002). Clinical outcomes and quality of life in elderly patients on peritoneal dialysis *vs.* hemodialysis. Peritoneal Dialysis International, 22, 463–470. Retrieved from http://www.ncbi.nlm.nih.gov/pubmed/12322817

Hays, R. D., Kallich, J. D., Mapes, D. L., Coons, S. J., & Carter, W. B. (1994). Development of the Kidney Disease Quality of Life (KDQOL^{TM}) Instrument. Quality of Life Research, 3, 329–338. doi:10.1007/BF00451725

Hicks, L. S., Cleary, P. D., Epstein, A. M., & Ayanian, J. Z. (2004). Differences in health-related quality of life and treatment preferences among Black and White patients with end-stage renal disease. Quality of Life Research, 13, 1129–1138. doi:10.1023/B:QURE.0000031350.56924.cc

Higginson, I. J., & Carr, A. J. (2001). Measuring quality of life: Using quality of life measures in the clinical setting. British Medical Journal, 322, 1297–1300. doi:10.1136/bmj.322.7297.1297

Hinrichsen, G. A., Lieberman, J. A., Pollack, S., & Steinberg, H. (1989). Depression in hemodialysis patients. Psychosomatics, 30, 284–289. doi:10.1016/S0033-3182(89)72273-8

Holley, J. L., & Nespor, S. (1994). An analysis of factors affecting employment of chronic dialysis patients. American Journal of Kidney Diseases, 23, 681–685. Retrieved from http://www.ncbi.nlm.nih.gov/pubmed/8172210

Hsieh, R.-L., & Lee, W.-C. (2007). Does exercise training during hemodialysis really improve dialysis efficacy? Archives of Physical Medicine and Rehabilitation, 88, 130. doi:10.1016/j.apmr.2006.11.008

Ifudu, O., Dawood, M., Homel, P., & Friedman, E. A. (1996). Excess morbidity in patients starting uremia therapy without prior care by a nephrologist. American Journal of Kidney Diseases, 28, 841–845. doi:10.1016/S0272-6386(96)90383-2

Jang, E.-J., & Kim, H.-S. (2009). Effects of exercise intervention on physical fitness and health-relalted quality of life in hemodialysis patients. Journal of Korean Academy of Nursing, 39, 584–593. doi:10.4040/jkan.2009.39.4.584

Jhamb, M., Pike, F., Ramer, S., Argyropoulos, C., Steel, J., Dew, M. A., Weisbord, S. D., *et al.* (2011). Impact of fatigue on outcomes in the hemodialysis (HEMO) study. American Journal of Nephrology, 33, 515–523. doi:10.1159/000328004

Kalantar-Zadeh, K., Kopple, J. D., Block, G., & Humphreys, M. H. (2001). Association among SF36 quality of life measures and nutrition, hospitalization, and mortality in hemodialysis. Journal of the American Society of Nephrology, 12, 2797–2806. Retrieved from http://www.ncbi.nlm.nih.gov/pubmed/11729250

Kao, T.-W., Lai, M.-S., Tsai, T.-J., Jan, C.-F., Chie, W.-C., & Chen, W.-Y. (2009). Economic, social, and psychological factors associated with health-related quality of life of chronic hemodialysis patients in northern Taiwan: A multicenter study. Artificial Organs, 33, 61–68. doi:10.1111/j.1525-1594.2008.00675.x

Kimmel, P. L. (2000). Just whose quality of life is it anyway? Controversies and consistencies in measurements of quality of life. Kidney International, 57, 113–120. doi:10.1046/j.1523-1755.2000.07419.x

Kimmel, P. L., Peterson, R. A., Weihs, K. L., Simmens, S. J., Boyle, D. H., Cruz, I., Umana, W. O., et al. (1995). Aspects of quality of life in hemodialysis patients. Journal of the American Society of Nephrology, 6, 1418–1426. Retrieved from http://www.ncbi.nlm.nih.gov/pubmed/8589317

Kimmel, P. L., Thamer, M., Richard, C. M., & Ray, N. F. (1998). Psychiatric illness in patients with end-stage renal disease. The American Journal of Medicine, 105, 214–221. doi:10.1016/S0002-9343(98)00245-9

Kimmel, P. L., Weihs, K. L., & Peterson, R. A. (1993). Survival in hemodialysis patients: the role of depression. Journal of the American Society of Nephrology, 4, 12–27. Retrieved from http://jasn.asnjournals.org/content/4/1/12.short

Kliger, A. S., & Finkelstein, F. O. (2009). Can we improve the quality of life for dialysis patients? American Journal of Kidney Diseases, 54, 993–995. doi:10.1053/j.ajkd.2009.09.005

Korevaar, J. C., Merkus, M. P., Jansen, M. A. M., Dekker, F. W., Boeschoten, E. W., & Krediet, R. T. (2002). Validation of the KDQOL-SF: A dialysis-targeted health measure. Quality of Life Research, 11, 437–447. doi:10.1023/A:1015631411960

Kovacs, A. Z., Molnar, M. Z., Szeifert, L., Ambrus, C., Molnar-Varga, M., Szentkiralyi, A., Mucsi, I., et al. (2011). Sleep disorders, depressive symptoms and health-related quality of life--a cross-sectional comparison between kidney transplant recipients and waitlisted patients on maintenance dialysis. Nephrology, Dialysis, Transplantation, 26, 1058–1065. doi:10.1093/ndt/gfq476

Krespi, R., Bone, M., Ahmad, R., Worthington, B., & Salmon, P. (2004). Haemodialysis patients' beliefs about renal failure and its treatment. Patient Education and Counseling, 53, 189–196. doi:10.1016/S0738-3991(03)00147-2

Kusztal, M., Nowak, K., Magott-Procelewska, M., Weyde, W., & Penar, J. (2003). Evaluation of health-related quality of life in dialysis patients. Personal experience using questionnaire SF-36. Polski Merkuriusz Lekarski, 14, 113–117. Retrieved from http://www.ncbi.nlm.nih.gov/pubmed/12728668

Kutner, N. G. (2004). Quality of life and daily hemodialysis. Seminars in Dialysis, 17, 92–98. doi:10.1111/j.0894-0959.2004.17203.x

Kutner, N. G., Zhang, R., & Brogan, D. (2005). Race, gender, and incident dialysis patients' reported health status and quality of life. Journal of the American Society of Nephrology, 16, 1440–1448. doi:10.1681/ASN.2004080639

Kutner, N. G., Zhang, R., & McClellan, W. M. (2000). Patient-reported quality of life early in dialysis treatment: Effects associated with usual exercise activity. Nephrology Nursing Journal, 27, 357–367. Retrieved from http://www.ncbi.nlm.nih.gov/pubmed/11276627

Lacson, E., Xu, J., Lin, S.-F., Dean, S. G., Lazarus, J. M., & Hakim, R. M. (2009). Association between achievement of hemodialysis quality-of-care indicators and quality-of-life scores. American Journal of Kidney Diseases, 54, 1098–1107. doi:10.1053/j.ajkd.2009.07.017

Lamping, D. L., Constantinovici, N., Roderick, P. J., Normand, C., Henderson, L. M., Harris, S. A. C., Brown, E. A., *et al.* (2000). Clinical outcomes, quality of life, and costs in the North Thames dialysis study of elderly people on dialysis: A prospective cohort study. The Lancet, 356, 1543–1550. doi:10.1016/S0140-6736(00)03123-8

Landreneau, K., Lee, K., & Landreneau, M. D. (2010). Quality of life in patients undergoing hemodialysis and renal transplantation--a meta-analytic review. Nephrology Nursing Journal, 37, 37–44. Retrieved from http://www.ncbi.nlm.nih.gov/pubmed/20333902

Laupacis, A., Muirhead, N., Keown, P., & Wong, C. (1992). A disease-specific questionnaire for assessing quality of life in patients on hemodialysis. Nephron, 60, 302–306. doi:10.1159/000186769

Leggat, J., Orzol, S., Hulbert-Shearon, T., Golper, T., Jones, C., Held, P., & Port, F. K. (1998). Noncompliance in hemodialysis: Predictors and survival analysis. American Journal of Kidney Diseases, 32, 139–145. doi:10.1053/ajkd.1998.v32.pm9669435

Lew, S. Q., & Piraino, B. (2005). Quality of life and psychological issues in peritoneal dialysis patients. Seminars in Dialysis, 18, 119–123. doi:10.1111/j.1525-139X.2005.18215.x

Lew-Starowicz, M., & Gellert, R. (2009). The sexuality and quality of life of hemodialyzed patients--ASED multicenter study. Palliative Medicine, 6, 1062–1071. doi:10.1111/j.1743-6109.2008.01040.x

Liem, Y. S., Bosch, J. L., Arends, L. R., Heijenbrok-Kal, M. H., & Hunink, M. G. M. (2007). Quality of life assessed with the Medical Outcomes Study Short Form 36-Item Health Survey of patients on renal replacement therapy: a systematic review and meta-analysis. Value in Health, 10, 390–397. doi:10.1111/j.1524-4733.2007.00193.x

Liem, Y. S., Bosch, J. L., & Hunink, M. G. M. (2008). Preference-based quality of life of patients on renal replacement therapy: A systematic review and meta-analysis. Value in Health, 11, 733–741. doi:10.1111/j.1524-4733.2007.00308.x

Lii, Y.-C., Tsay, S.-L., & Wang, T.-J. (2007). Group intervention to improve quality of life in haemodialysis patients. Journal of Clinical Nursing, 16, 268–275. doi:10.1111/j.1365-2702.2007.01963.x

Lo, C., Li, L., Lo, W., Chan, M., So, E., Tang, S., Yuen, M., *et al.* (1998). Benefits of exercise training in patients on continuous ambulatory peritoneal dialysis. American Journal of Kidney Diseases, 32, 1011–1018. Retrieved from http://www.ncbi.nlm.nih.gov/pubmed/9856517

Loos, C., Briançon, S., Frimat, L., Hanesse, B., & Kessler, M. (2003). Effect of end-stage renal disease on the quality of life of older patients. Journal of the American Geriatrics Society, 51, 229–233. doi:10.1046/j.1532-5415.2003.51062.x

Loos-Ayav, C., Frimat, L., Kessler, M., Chanliau, J., Durand, P.-Y., & Briançon, S. (2008). Changes in health-related quality of life in patients of self-care *vs.* in-center dialysis during the first year. Quality of Life Research, 17, 1–9. doi:10.1007/s11136-007-9286-1

Lopes, A. A., Bragg-Gresham, J. L., Goodkin, D. A., Fukuhara, S., Mapes, D. L., Young, E. W., Gillespie, B. W., *et al.* (2007). Factors associated with health-related quality of life among hemodialysis patients in the DOPPS. Quality of Life Research, 16, 545–557. doi:10.1007/s11136-006-9143-7

Low, J., Smith, G., Burns, A., & Jones, L. (2008). The impact of end-stage kidney disease (ESKD) on close persons: A literature review. Nephrology, Dialysis, Transplantation Plus, 1, 67–79. doi:10.1093/ndtplus/sfm046

Lowrie, E. G., Curtin, R. B., LePain, N., & Schatell, D. (2003). Medical outcomes study short form-36: A consistent and powerful predictor of morbidity and mortality in dialysis patients. American Journal of Kidney Diseases, 41, 1286–1292. doi:10.1016/S0272-6386(03)00361-5

Maglakelidze, N., Pantsulaia, T., Tchokhonelidze, I., Managadze, L., & Chkhotua, A. (2011). Assessment of health-related quality of life in renal transplant recipients and dialysis patients. Transplantation Proceedings, 43, 376–379. doi:10.1016/j.transproceed.2010.12.015

Manns, B. J., Walsh, M. W., Culleton, B. F., Hemmelgarn, B. R., Tonelli, M., Schorr, M., & Klarenbach, S. W. (2009). Nocturnal hemodialysis does not improve overall measures of quality of life compared to conventional hemodialysis. Kidney International, 75, 542–549. doi:10.1038/ki.2008.639

Mapes, D. L., Bragg-Gresham, J. L., Bommer, J., Fukuhara, S., McKevitt, P., Wikstrom, B., & Lopes, A. A. (2004). Health-related quality of life in the Dialysis Outcomes and Practice Patterns Study (DOPPS). American Journal of Kidney Diseases, 44, 54–60. doi:10.1053/j.ajkd.2004.08.012

Martin, C. R., & Thompson, D. R. (2000). Prediction of quality of life in patients with end-stage renal disease. British Journal of Health Psychology, 5, 41–55. doi:10.1348/135910700168757

Mau, L.-W., Chiu, H.-C., Chang, P.-Y., Hwang, S.-C., & Hwang, S.-J. (2008). Health-related quality of life of Taiwanese dialysis patients: Effects of dialysis modality. The Kaohsiung Journal of Medical Sciences, 24, 453–460. doi:10.1016/S1607-551X(09)70002-6

McFarlane, P. A., Bayoumi, A. M., Pierratos, A., & Redelmeier, D. A. (2003). The quality of life and cost utility of home nocturnal and conventional in-center hemodialysis. Kidney International, 64, 1004–1011. doi:10.1046/j.1523-1755.2003.00157.x

Mendelssohn, D. C., Mullaney, S. R., Jung, B., Blake, P. G., & Mehta, R. L. (2001). What do American nephrologists think about dialysis modality selection? American Journal of Kidney Diseases, 37, 22–29. doi:10.1053/ajkd.2001.20635

Merkus, M. P., Jager, K. J., Dekker, F. W., Boeschoten, E. W., Stevens, P. E., & Krediet, R. T. (1997). Quality of life in patients on chronic dialysis: Self-assessment 3 months after the start of treatment. American Journal of Kidney Diseases, 29, 584–592. doi:10.1016/S0272-6386(97)90342-5

Mingardi, G., Cornalba, L., Cortinovis, E., Ruggiata, R., Mosconi, P., & Apolone, G. (1999). Health-related quality of life in dialysis patients. A report from an Italian study using the SF-36 Health Survey. DIA-QOL Group. Nephrology, Dialysis, Transplantation, 14, 1503–1510. Retrieved from http://www.ncbi.nlm.nih.gov/pubmed/10383015

Mohr, P. E., Neumann, P. J., Franco, S. J., Marainen, J., Lockridge, R., & Ting, G. (2001). The case for daily dialysis: its impact on costs and quality of life. American Journal of Kidney Diseases, 37, 777–789. Retrieved from http://www.ncbi.nlm.nih.gov/pubmed/11273878

Moist, L. M., Bragg-Gresham, J. L., Pisoni, R. L., Saran, R., Akiba, T., Jacobson, S. H., Fukuhara, S., et al. (2008). Travel time to dialysis as a predictor of health-related quality of life, adherence, and mortality: the Dialysis Outcomes and Practice Patterns Study (DOPPS). American Journal of Kidney Diseases, 51, 641–650. doi:10.1053/j.ajkd.2007.12.021

Moreno, F., López-Gómez, J. M., Sanz-Guajardo, D., Jofré, R., & Valderrábano, F. (1996). Quality of life in dialysis patients. A Spanish multicentre study. Nephrology Dialysis Transplantation, 11, 125–129. doi:10.1093/ndt/11.supp2.125

Morsch, C. M., Gonçalves, L. F., & Barros, E. J. G. (2006). Health-related quality of life among haemodialysis patients--relationship with clinical indicators, morbidity and mortality. Journal of Clinical Nursing, 15, 498–504. doi:10.1111/j.1365-2702.2006.01349.x

Mujais, S. K., Story, K., Brouillette, J., Takano, T., Soroka, S., Franek, C., Mendelssohn, D. C., *et al.* (2009). Health-related quality of life and hemoglobin levels in chronic kidney disease patients. Clinical Journal of the American Society of Nephrology, 4, 33–38. doi:10.2215/CJN.00630208

Mustata, S., Cooper, L., Langrick, N., Simon, N., Jassal, S. V., & Oreopoulos, D. G. (2005). The effect of a Tai Chi exercise program on quality of life in patients on peritoneal dialysis: A pilot study. Peritoneal Dialysis International, 25, 291–294. Retrieved from http://www.ncbi.nlm.nih.gov/pubmed/15981780

Niu, S.-F., & Li, I.-C. (2005). Quality of life of patients having renal replacement therapy. Journal of Advanced Nursing, 51, 15–21. doi:10.1111/j.1365-2648.2005.03455.x

Ohri-Vachaspati, P., & Sehgal, A. R. (1999). Quality of life implications of inadequate protein nutrition among hemodialysis patients. Journal of Renal Nutrition, 9, 9–13. doi:10.1016/S1051-2276(99)90016-X

Painter, P., Carlson, L., Carey, S., Paul, S. M., & Myll, J. (2000a). Physical functioning and health-related quality-of-life changes with exercise training in hemodialysis patients. American Journal of Kidney Diseases, 35, 482–492. doi:10.1016/S0272-6386(00)70202-2

Painter, P., Carlson, L., Carey, S., Paul, S. M., & Myll, J. (2000b). Low-functioning hemodialysis patients improve with exercise training. American Journal of Kidney Diseases, 36, 600–608. doi:10.1053/ajkd.2000.16200

Parsons, T. L., Toffelmire, E. B., & King-VanVlack, C. E. (2006). Exercise training during hemodialysis improves dialysis efficacy and physical performance. Archives of Physical Medicine and Rehabilitation, 87, 680–687. doi:10.1016/j.apmr.2005.12.044

Patrick, D. L., & Deyo, R. A. (1989). Generic and disease-specific measures in assessing health status and quality of life. Medical Care, 27, S217–S232. Retrieved from http://www.ncbi.nlm.nih.gov/pubmed/2646490

Peng, Y.-S., Chiang, C.-K., Hung, K.-Y., Chang, C.-H., Lin, C.-Y., Yang, C.-S., Chen, T.-W., *et al.* (2010). Are both psychological and physical dimensions in health-related quality of life associated with mortality in hemodialysis patients: A 7-year Taiwan cohort study. Blood Purification, 30, 98–105. doi:10.1159/000319002

Peterson, R. A., Kimmel, P. L., Sacks, C. R., Mesquita, M. L., Simmens, S. J., & Reiss, D. (1991). Depression, perception of illness and mortality in patients with end-stage renal disease. International Journal of Psychiatry in Medicine, 21, 343–354. Retrieved from http://www.ncbi.nlm.nih.gov/pubmed/1774125

Plantinga, L. C., Fink, N. E., Harrington-Levey, R., Finkelstein, F. O., Hebah, N., Powe, N. R., & Jaar, B. G. (2010). Association of social support with outcomes in incident dialysis patients. Clinical Journal of the American Society of Nephrology, 5, 1480–1488. doi:10.2215/CJN.01240210

Plantinga, L. C., Fink, N. E., Jaar, B. G., Huang, I.-C., Wu, A. W., Meyer, K. B., & Powe, N. R. (2007). Relation between level or change of hemoglobin and generic and disease-specific quality of life measures in hemodialysis. Quality of Life Research, 16, 755–765. doi:10.1007/s11136-007-9176-6

Porter, A. C., Fischer, M. J., Brooks, D., Bruce, M., Charleston, J., Cleveland, W. H., Dowie, D., *et al.* (2012). Quality of life and psychosocial factors in African Americans with hypertensive chronic kidney disease. Translational Research, 159, 4–11. doi:10.1016/j.trsl.2011.09.004

Pucheu, S., Consoli, S. M., D'Auzac, C., Français, P., & Issad, B. (2004). Do health causal attributions and coping strategies act as moderators of quality of life in peritoneal dialysis patients? Journal of Psychosomatic Research, 56, 317–322. doi:10.1016/S0022-3999(03)00080-1

Pugh-Clarke, K., Naish, P. F., & Mercer, T. M. (2006). Quality of life in chronic kidney disease. Journal of Renal Care, 32, 156–159. doi:10.1111/j.1755-6686.2006.tb00010.x

Rabindranath, K. S., Adams, J., Ali, T. Z., Daly, C., Vale, L., & Macleod, A. M. (2007). Automated *vs.* continuous ambulatory peritoneal dialysis: A systematic review of randomized controlled trials. Nephrology, Dialysis, Transplantation, 22, 2991–2998. doi:10.1093/ndt/gfm515

Rabindranath, K. S., Strippoli, G. F. M., Daly, C., Roderick, P. J., Wallace, S. A., & Macleod, A. M. (2006). Haemodiafiltration, haemofiltration and haemodialysis for end-stage kidney disease. Cochrane Database of Systematic Reviews, CD006258. doi:10.1002/14651858.CD006258

Rambod, M., Shabani, M., Shokrpour, N., Rafii, F., & Mohammadalliha, J. (2011). Quality of life of hemodialysis and renal transplantation patients. The Health Care Manager, 30, 23–28. doi:10.1097/HCM.0b013e3182078ab6

Ramirez, S. P., Macêdo, D. S., Sales, P. M. G., Figueiredo, S. M., Daher, E. F., Araújo, S. M., Pargament, K. I., *et al.* (2012). The relationship between religious coping, psychological distress and quality of life in hemodialysis patients. Journal of Psychosomatic Research, 72, 129–135. doi:10.1016/j.jpsychores.2011.11.012

Rayment, G. A., & Bonner, A. (2008). Daily dialysis: Exploring the impact for patients and nurses. International Journal of Nursing Practice, 14, 221–227. doi:10.1111/j.1440-172X.2008.00690.x

Reboredo, M. D. M., Henrique, D. M. N., Faria, R. D. S., Chaoubah, A., Bastos, M. G., & De Paula, R. B. (2010). Exercise training during hemodialysis reduces blood pressure and increases physical functioning and quality of life. Artificial Organs, 34, 586–593. doi:10.1111/j.1525-1594.2009.00929.x

Ross, E. a, Hollen, T. L., & Fitzgerald, B. M. (2006). Observational study of an Arts-in-Medicine Program in an outpatient hemodialysis unit. American Journal of Kidney Diseases, 47, 462–468. doi:10.1053/j.ajkd.2005.11.030

Roumelioti, M.-E., Wentz, A., Schneider, M. F., Gerson, A. C., Hooper, S. R., Benfield, M., Warady, B. A., *et al.* (2010). Sleep and fatigue symptoms in children and adolescents with CKD: a cross-sectional analysis from the chronic kidney disease in children (CKiD) study. American Journal of Kidney Diseases, 55, 269–280. doi:10.1053/j.ajkd.2009.09.021

Saban, K. L., Stroupe, K. T., Bryant, F. B., Reda, D. J., Browning, M. M., & Hynes, D. M. (2008). Comparison of health-related quality of life measures for chronic renal failure: Quality of well-being scale, short-form-6D, and the kidney disease quality of life instrument. Quality of Life Research, 17, 1103–1115. doi:10.1007/s11136-008-9387-5

Sacks, C. R., Peterson, R. A., & Kimmel, P. L. (1990). Perception of illness and depression in chronic renal disease. American Journal of Kidney Diseases, 15, 31–39. Retrieved from http://www.ncbi.nlm.nih.gov/pubmed/2294731

Santos, P. R., Daher, E. F., Silva, G. B., Libório, A. B., & Kerr, L. R. (2009). Quality of life assessment among haemodialysis patients in a single centre: A 2-year follow-up. Quality of Life Research, 18, 541–546. doi:10.1007/s11136-009-9474-2

Saran, R., Bragg-Gresham, J. L., Rayner, H. C., Goodkin, D. a, Keen, M. L., Van Dijk, P. C., Kurokawa, K., et al. (2003). Nonadherence in hemodialysis: associations with mortality, hospitalization, and practice patterns in the DOPPS. Kidney international, 64, 254–62. doi:10.1046/j.1523-1755.2003.00064.x

Sareen, J., Jacobi, F., Cox, B. J., Belik, S.-L., Clara, I., & Stein, M. B. (2006). Disability and poor quality of life associated with comorbid anxiety disorders and physical conditions. Archives of Internal Medicine, 166, 2109–2116. doi:10.1001/archinte.166.19.2109

Sathvik, B. S., Parthasarathi, G., Narahari, M. G., & Gurudev, K. C. (2008). An assessment of the quality of life in hemodialysis patients using the WHOQOL-BREF questionnaire. Indian Journal of Nephrology, 18, 141–149. doi:10.4103/0971-4065.45288

Sayin, A., Mutluay, R., & Sindel, S. (2007). Quality of life in hemodialysis, peritoneal dialysis, and transplantation patients. Transplantation Proceedings, 39, 3047–3053. doi:10.1016/j.transproceed.2007.09.030

Sesso, R., Rodrigues-Neto, J. F., & Ferraz, M. B. (2003). Impact of socioeconomic status on the quality of life of ESRD patients. American Journal of Kidney Diseases, 41, 186–195. doi:10.1053/ajkd.2003.50003

Singer, P. A., Martin, D. K., & Kelner, M. (1999). Quality end-of-life care: Patients' perspectives. Journal of the American Medical Association, 281, 163–168. doi:10.1001/jama.281.2.163

Spiegel, B. M. R., Melmed, G., Robbins, S., & Esrailian, E. (2008). Biomarkers and health-related quality of life in end-stage renal disease: A systematic review. Clinical Journal of the American Society of Nephrology, 3, 1759–1768. doi:10.2215/CJN.00820208

Stojanovic, M., Ilic, S., & Stefanovic, V. (2006). Influence of co-morbidity on health-related quality of life in patients treated with hemodialysis. The International Journal of Artifical Organs, 29, 1053–1061. Retrieved from http://www.ncbi.nlm.nih.gov/pubmed/17160962

Su, C.-Y., Lu, X.-H., Chen, W., & Wang, T. (2009). Promoting self-management improves the health status of patients having peritoneal dialysis. Journal of Advanced Nursing, 65, 1381–1389. doi:10.1111/j.1365-2648.2009.04993.x

Taskapan, H., Ates, F., Kaya, B., Emul, M., Kaya, M., Taskapan, C., & Sahin, I. (2005). Psychiatric disorders and large interdialytic weight gain in patients on chronic haemodialysis. Nephrology, 10, 15–20. doi:10.1111/j.1440-1797.2005.00321.x

Tawney, K. W., Tawney, P. J. W., Hladik, G., Hogan, S. L., Falk, R. J., Weaver, C., Moore, D. T., et al. (2000). The life readiness program: A physical rehabilitation program for patients on hemodialysis. American Journal of Kidney Diseases, 36, 581–591. doi:10.1053/ajkd.2000.16197

Theofilou, P. (2012). Quality of life and mental health in hemodialysis and peritoneal dialysis patients: the role of health beliefs. International Urology and Nephrology, 44, 245–253. doi:10.1007/s11255-011-9975-0

Thong, M. S. Y., Van Dijk, S., Noordzij, M., Boeschoten, E. W., Krediet, R. T., Dekker, F. W., & Kaptein, A. A. (2009). Symptom clusters in incident dialysis patients: Associations with clinical variables and quality of life. Nephrology, Dialysis, Transplantation, 24, 225–230. doi:10.1093/ndt/gfn449

Timmers, L., Thong, M. S. Y., Dekker, F. W., Boeschoten, E. W., Heijmans, M., Rijken, M., Weinman, J., et al. (2008). Illness perceptions in dialysis patients and their association with quality of life. Psychology & Health, 23, 679–690. doi:10.1080/14768320701246535

Tovbin, D., Gidron, Y., Jean, T., Granovsky, R., & Schnieder, A. (2003). Relative importance and interrelations between psychosocial factors and individualized quality of life of hemodialysis patients. Quality of Life Research, 12, 709–717. doi:10.1023/A:1025101601822

Tsai, Y.-C., Hung, C.-C., Hwang, S.-J., Wang, S.-L., Hsiao, S.-M., Lin, M.-Y., Kung, L.-F., et al. (2010). Quality of life predicts risks of end-stage renal disease and mortality in patients with chronic kidney disease. Nephrology, Dialysis, Transplantation, 25, 1621–1626. doi:10.1093/ndt/gfp671

Tsay, S.-L., Lee, Y.-C., & Lee, Y.-C. (2005). Effects of an adaptation training programme for patients with end-stage renal disease. Journal of Advanced Nursing, 50, 39–46. doi:10.1111/j.1365-2648.2004.03347.x

Tsevat, J., Dawson, N. V., Wu, A. W., Lynn, J., Soukup, J. R., Cook, F., Vidaillet, H., et al. (1998). Health values of hospitalized patients 80 years or older. Journal of the American Medical Association, 279, 371–375. doi:10.1001/jama.279.5.371

Tsevat, J., Weeks, J. C., Guadagnoli, E., Tosteson, A. N. A., Mangione, C. M., Pliskin, J. S., Weinstein, M. C., et al. (1994). Using health-related quality-of-life information: Clinical encounters, clinical trials, and health policy. Journal of General Internal Medicine, 9, 576–582. Retrieved from http://www.ncbi.nlm.nih.gov/pubmed/7823230

Tucker, C. M., Ziller, R. C., Smith, W. R., Mars, D. R., & Coons, M. P. (1991). Quality of life of patients on in-center hemodialysis vs. continuous ambulatory peritoneal dialysis. Peritoneal Dialysis International, 11, 341–346. Retrieved from http://www.ncbi.nlm.nih.gov/pubmed/1751601

Unruh, M. L., Benz, R., Greene, T., Yan, G., Beddhu, S., DeVita, M., Dwyer, J. T., et al. (2004). Effects of hemodialysis dose and membrane flux on health-related quality of life in the HEMO Study. Kidney International, 66, 355–366. doi:10.1111/j.1523-1755.2004.00738.x

Valderrábano, F., Jofré, R., & López-Gómez, J. M. (2001). Quality of life in end-stage renal disease patients. American Journal of Kidney Diseases, 38, 443–464. doi:10.1053/ajkd.2001.26824

Vale, L., Cody, J., Wallace, S. A., Daly, C., Campbell, M., Grant, A., Khan, I. H., et al. (2004). Continuous ambulatory peritoneal dialysis (CAPD) vs. hospital or home haemodialysis for end-stage renal disease in adults. Cochrane Database of Systematic Reviews, CD003963. doi:10.1002/14651858.CD003963.pub2

Van Eps, C. L., Jeffries, J. K., Johnson, D. W., Campbell, S. B., Isbel, N. M., Mudge, D. W., & Hawley, C. M. (2010). Quality of life and alternate nightly nocturnal home hemodialysis. Hemodialysis International, 14, 29–38. doi:10.1111/j.1542-4758.2009.00419.x

Vos, P. F., Zilch, O., & Kooistra, M. P. (2001). Clinical outcome of daily dialysis. American Journal of Kidney Diseases, 37, S99–S102. doi:10.1053/ajkd.2001.20761

Wang, W., Tonelli, M., Hemmelgarn, B. R., Gao, S., Johnson, J. A., Taub, K., & Manns, B. J. (2008). The effect of increasing dialysis dose in overweight hemodialysis patients on quality of life: a 6-week randomized crossover trial. American Journal of Kidney Diseases, 51, 796–803. doi:10.1053/j.ajkd.2007.12.031

Ware, Jr., J. E., & Sherbourne, C. D. (1992). The MOS 36-item short-form health survey (SF-36). I. Conceptual framework and item selection. Medical Care, 30, 473–483. doi:10.1097/00005650-199206000-00002

Wasserfallen, J.-B., Halabi, G., Saudan, P., Perneger, T., Feldman, H. I., Martin, P.-Y., & Wauters, J.-P. (2004). Quality of life on chronic dialysis: Comparison between haemodialysis and peritoneal dialysis. Nephrology, Dialysis, Transplantation, 19, 1594–1599. doi:10.1093/ndt/gfh175

White, C. A., Pilkey, R. M., Lam, M., & Holland, D. C. (2002). Pre-dialysis clinic attendance improves quality of life among hemodialysis patients. BMC Nephrology, 3. doi:10.1186/1471-2369/3/3

Wiedebusch, S., Konrad, M., Foppe, H., Reichwald-Klugger, E., Schaefer, F., Schreiber, V., & Muthny, F. A. (2010). Health-related quality of life, psychosocial strains, and coping in parents of children with chronic renal failure. Pediatric Nephrology, 25, 1477–1485. doi:10.1007/s00467-010-1540-z

Williams, A. W., Chebrolu, S. B., Ing, T. S., Ting, G., Blagg, C. R., Twardowski, Z. J., Woredekal, Y., *et al.* (2004). Early clinical, quality-of-life, and biochemical changes of "daily hemodialysis" (6 dialyses per week). American Journal of Kidney Diseases, 43, 90–102. doi:10.1053/j.ajkd.2003.09.017

Wingard, R. L., Pupim, L. B., Krishnan, M., Shintani, A., Ikizler, T. A., & Hakim, R. M. (2007). Early intervention improves mortality and hospitalization rates in incident hemodialysis patients: RightStart program. Clinical Journal of the American Society of Nephrology, 2, 1170–1175. doi:10.2215/CJN.04261206

Wiser, N. A., Shane, J. M., McGuigan, A. T., Memken, J. A., & Olsson, P. J. (1997). The effects of a group nutrition education program on nutrition knowledge, nutrition status, and quality of life in hemodialysis patients. Journal of Renal Nutrition, 7, 187–193. doi:10.1016/S1051-2276(97)90017-0

Wu, A. W., Fink, N. E., Marsh-Manzi, J. V. R., Meyer, K. B., Finkelstein, F. O., Chapman, M. M., & Powe, N. R. (2004). Changes in quality of life during hemodialysis and peritoneal dialysis treatment: Generic and disease specific measures. Journal of the American Society of Nephrology, 15, 743–753. doi:10.1097/01.ASN.0000113315.81448.CA

Yarlas, A. S., White, M. K., Yang, M., Saris-Baglama, R. N., Bech, P. G., & Christensen, T. (2011). Measuring the health status burden in hemodialysis patients using the SF-36® health survey. Quality of Life Research, 20, 383–389. doi:10.1007/s11136-010-9764-8

Yokoyama, Y., Suzukamo, Y., Hotta, O., Yamazaki, S., Kawaguchi, T., Hasegawa, T., Chiba, S., *et al.* (2009). Dialysis staff encouragement and fluid control adherence in patients on hemodialysis. Nephrology Nursing Journal, 36, 289–297. Retrieved from http://www.ncbi.nlm.nih.gov/pubmed/19588696

Zabel, R., Ash, S., King, N., Juffs, P., & Bauer, J. (2012). Relationships between appetite and quality of life in hemodialysis patients. Appetite, 59, 194–199. doi:10.1016/j.appet.2012.02.016

CHAPTER 5

Quality of Life Assessment in Kidney Transplantation

Pavlos Malindretos[1,*], Stamatina. Zili[2] and Pantelis Sarafidis[3]

[1]Department of Nephrology, Peritoneal Dialysis Section, Achillopouleion General Hospital, Volos, Greece; [2]Department of Internal Medicine, Papageorgiou General Hospital, Thessaloniki and [3]1st Medical Department, Aristotle University, Thessaloniki, Greece

Abstract: Transplanted patients generally experience lower health related quality of life (HRQoL) compared to general population. The vast majority of studies evaluating quality of life of patients before and after renal transplantation are in favour of transplanted patients. Immunosuppressive treatment side effects seem to have a negative impact on patients' HRQoL. Nevertheless, HRQoL is generally significantly improved in children, adolescents and adults alike. Further more, living kidney transplant donors seem to present better HRQoL and improved depression status after a successful kidney transplantation. Even when older living donors are carefully selected, there is no need to be excluded from transplantation screening programs. Kidney transplantation represents the only known definite treatment of end - stage kidney disease (ESKD). When carefully planned and performed it will lead to both improved survival and health related quality of life of patients with advanced chronic kidney disease.

Keywords: Health related quality of life, HRQoL, quality of life, QoL, transplantation, kidney transplantation, children, adolescents, adults.

QOL ASSESSMENT IN KIDNEY TRANSPLANTATION

Transplanted patients generally experience lower health - related quality of life (HRQoL) compared to general population. Compared to heart and liver, kidney transplant recipients seem to have lower HRQoL in the long run (Karam *et al.*, 2003). Probably this could be attributed at least in part to medication side effects and dietary restrictions. In the following pages lies a narrative review which aims to present to the reader as many different approaches as possible regarding correlation between kidney transplantation and health related quality of life. An

Address correspondence to Pavlos Malindretos: Department of Nephrology, Peritoneal Dialysis Section, Achillopouleion General Hospital, Volos, Greece; Tel: 00306937445545; Fax: 00302421351262; E-mail: pavlosmm@hotmail.com

additional effort was made so that quality of life (QoL) of children and adults, living relative and non - relative donors, men and women would be incorporated in the manuscript.

HRQOL INSTRUMENTS AND KIDNEY TRANSPLANTATION

Various attempts have been made in order to develop and validate quality of life instruments in kidney transplanted patients (Gentile *et al.*, 2008). Identifying factors are in general similar to those recognized in chronic kidney disease patients. Among them, physical health, mental health, medical care, fear of losing the graft, and treatment seem to be major determinants.

As it has been already indicated in a previous chapter, HRQoL measurement instruments usually comprise two distinct parts. Generic instruments consist of general questions and can be applied in healthy individuals as well. On the other hand, disease specific instruments target at specific symptoms that are common to a disease or condition. Most commonly used questionnaires are: Short Form 36 (SF-36) (Hays *et al.*, 1996), Sickness Impact Profile (Gilson *et al.*, 1975), and Beck Depression Inventory (Beck *et al.*, 1961). All of them comprise various questions aiming at physical, social, emotional and mental health. A great number of these instruments have been developed and applied by the researchers, aiming mainly at a specific determinant or part of HRQoL. For example, in order to answer to the question: "what is caregivers' perception of patients HRQoL?" (Molzahn *et al.*, 1997), or in order to estimate depression status in various conditions (Beck *et al.*, 1961). Regardless, they have all been validated in order to reflect a true difference in all major components of HRQoL when such a difference exists.

HRQOL IN KIDNEY TRANSPLANTATION - INSTRUMENT IMPLEMENTATION

But, let's start from the very beginning. Are patients influenced just from their presence in a "waiting list?" Being in waiting-list for renal or other organ transplantation represents by itself a significant psychological pressor factor for these patients. An appealing approach would suggest that end-stage renal disease patients frequently are receiving dialysis (peritoneal or hemodialysis) treatment and thus are subject to significant dietary restrictions. For example, potassium containing aliments (*e.g.,* fruits) and phosphate containing foods (like meat products, milk products, *etc.*) are restricted (Kalantar - Zadeh *et al.,* 2002). Moreover, patients on dialysis are subjected to liquids consumption restriction, including water consumption (Tovazzi *et al.,* 2012; Kugler *et al.,* 2011), since their urine quantity (if any) is diminished. This restriction is represented by inter-dialytic weight gain, which represents the weight gained between two consecutive dialysis sessions. Additionally, they are obligated to consume a large number of different pills daily in order to maintain an acceptable health status (Mason, 2011; Lam *et al.,* 2010). And as if these were not enough, they are subjected to a periodic dialysis program three times a week. There are various limitations to the simplistic assumption that dialysis patients on kidney transplant waiting list have better quality of life. To start with, treating doctors inevitably chose patients in good general condition to be candidates for transplantation. Additionally, even if we suppose that patients are perfectly matched regarding age, sex, annual income, family status and presence of comorbid conditions, still it should be taken into consideration the fact that patients willing to receive an allograft most probably are more optimistic regarding their future and as a consequence less depressed. On the other hand, even if so, making an effort to prepare and incorporate more patients to the waiting list could improve their quality of life and depression status.

In accordance with these, investigators have observed that patients not waiting for renal transplantation are generally older, are more likely to have diabetes and hypertension; and present increased mortality. And as expected, they present lower scores in the major dimensions of quality of life, including functional capacity, physical limitation, pain, social life, role emotional and mental health (Santos, 2011).

Studies evaluating prospectively quality of life of patients before and after renal transplantation were in favor of transplanted patients (Dew *et al.,* 1997). A major improvement is observed in mental health, physical and functional components of health-related quality of life (Muehrer, & Becker, 2005).

Sleep disorders such as insomnia, sleep apnea syndrome and restless legs syndrome are common in end stage renal disease and transplanted patients. In a cross-sectional study aiming to assess fatigue and sleep quality before and after kidney transplantation, it was observed that pre-transplanted kidney disease patients had elevated levels of fatigue frequency, fatigue severity, and fatigue disruptiveness compared to post-transplanted ones. Additionally, it was observed that pre-transplanted patients experienced more difficulty with sleep quality, latency, duration, efficiency and disturbance (Rodrigue *et al.*, 2011).

It is worth mentioning that some investigators have observed better HRQoL in prevalent hemodialysis patients being on waiting list, even compared to those receiving a kidney transplant (Szeifert *et al.*, 2012). Fact which suggests that patients should be well informed and prepared, thus life with a donated kidney will not be frustrating.

On the other hand, there is data suggesting that donors' HRQoL might be negatively influenced by kidney donation (Chien *et al.*, 2010), thus implying that HRQoL of possible donors should be carefully evaluated before actual donation.

Treatment adverse effects expressed as skin diseases represent a significant stressor factor in kidney transplanted patients. Among them, dry skin, hypertrichosis, sebaceous gland hyperplasia, genital warts and frequent appearance of herpes simplex virus type I infections are among the most significant impact factors of HRQoL in kidney transplanted patients (Moloney *et al.*, 2005).

Immunosuppressive treatment has been incriminated for causing various adverse effects, leading in deteriorated health-related quality of life (HRQoL) and non-adherence to medication. Cyclosporine has been associated with cardiovascular, metabolic, periodontal and dermatological side effects. It has been observed that regardless from initial indication (either cardiovascular, or cosmetic), switching from cyclosporine to tacrolimus, improves disease-specific quality of life (Franke *et al.*, 2006). In transplanted patients from Canada has been observed that type of calcineurin inhibitor (CNI), either cyclosporine or tacrolimus doesn't seem to have a different impact on their quality of life, but patients preferred to continue on tacrolimus (Prasad *et al.*, 2010).

Non-adherence to immunosuppressant treatment even though present in adults, it is less frequent than the one observed in adolescents. Adults seem to be more concerned about lifestyle restrictions and as an example they would rather prefer to suppress the evening dose and follow a low-intensity treatment (Morales *et al.*, 2012).

Sexual dysfunction is quite common among female patients suffering from chronic kidney disease, affecting up to 60-70% of women on dialysis (Beck *et al.*, 1961). Furthermore, it has been observed that even though reduced sexual desire disorder might affect 100% of women on hemodialysis, it will affect 67% of those on peritoneal dialysis and only 31% of the transplanted females (Toorians *et al.*, 1997).

Is there any difference between living donor and diseased donor recipients? There is data suggesting that quality of life of diseased donor recipients decreased a few years after transplantation (Suzuki *et al.*, 2012).

Patients suffering from kidney disease present deteriorated health-related quality of life. Concomitant presence of another severe illness as cancer further reduces quality of life in chronic kidney disease, dialysis and kidney transplant recipients (Wong *et al.*, 2012).

Since renal function is one of the major determinants of quality of life, one would expect this correlation to be continued after kidney transplantation. Actually it has been observed that all health-related quality of life scales are inversely associated with chronic kidney disease following kidney transplantation (Neri *et al.*, 2011).

Kidney transplanted patients frequently experience voiding dysfunction and nocturia (Mitsui *et al.*, 2009). These bedside psychological factors, inevitably might affect HRQoL. Thus, lower urinary tract symptoms should be addressed properly in order to improve HRQoL of these patients.

Anemia is a known determinant of HRQoL in CKD patients. This is also valid for transplanted patients. Especially kidney transplanted patients with lower scores at physical and mental components are expected to benefit the most from hematocrit improvement (Kawada *et al.*, 2009). These findings offer the possibility to identify those patients who's HRQoL could be improved.

There have been various discussions regarding capability of older living kidney donors and whether they should be allowed to donate. Truth is that itra- and postoperative complication rates and early graft survival are not significantly different to that observed in younger donors (Minnee *et al.*, 2008). Additionally investigators have observed that older kidney donors have similar quality of life. Obviously, when older donors are carefully selected, there is no need to exclude them from transplantation screening programs.

Even though between genders, no significant differences are observed in transplanted patients, there are differences between them and healthy controls. Transplanted women seem to be significantly affected as regards their social activities, pain and general health. Transplanted men on the other hand, beside social activities, pain and general health, they also present diminished psycho-physical energy (Cornella *et al.*, 2008).

What is our perception of patients' HRQoL? It has been found that nurses rate patients' HRQoL significantly lower than patients rate themselves, while physicians rate them higher (Molzahn *et al.*, 1997).

As regards transplanted children (3 to 19 years old), it has been observed that they experience significantly higher levels of mental health problems and lower health-related quality of life compared to healthy controls. Body mass index and maximal oxygen uptake are among major determinants of their HRQoL and especially mental health (Diseth *et al.*, 2011). This reminds us of the ancient Greek proverb that "healthy mind resides in a healthy body", indicating that children rehabilitation after renal transplantation should focus on both physical activity and psychological state.

Restrictions that inevitably follow any organ transplantation, as well as adherence to medication, represent a major concern in adolescent renal transplant patients (Dobbels *et al.*, 2010). Adolescents rate their quality of life as satisfactory, but non-adherence to treatment is very frequent in this population. Depression symptoms are also frequent in adolescents. It seems that they are greatly affected by treatment side effects, like increased appetite, fatigue and headache. Mainly those factors affecting their external appearance, as hair loss, thinning of hair and warts on hands or feet (Dobbels *et al.*, 2010). Aberrant behavior is also noted in this subgroup of patients including smoking, illicit drug use, dietary non-adherence and suboptimal exercise levels.

Investigators seem to agree that HRQoL in pediatric population, regarding both physical and psychological domain, is better in transplanted compared to dialysis patients (Goldstein *et al.*, 2006).

HRQOL of transplanted children seems to be influenced by dialysis duration, young age at renal transplantation, living-related donation, steroid treatment, adverse family relationships and maternal distress (Falger *et al.*, 2008).

Regarding adolescent kidney transplant recipients, it is quite relieving that they have consistent and high values of HRQoL, reflecting their perception of being close to full health (Tong *et al.*, 2011).

Being a mother is the most sacred relationship in the world. There is data suggesting that living donor mothers improve their depression scores and their quality of life after kidney donation. Improvement in all domains is significantly greater than the one seen in donors with other relationships (Guleria *et al.*, 2011).

Before transplantation is freely suggested to all end stage renal disease patients, it should be kept in mind that significant treatment transitions might lead to significant changes of HRQoL. Whilst a successful transplantation will lead to HRQoL improvement, transplantation failure might lead to significant deterioration of HRQoL post transplant (Griva *et al.*, 2012).

CONCLUSIONS

All things considered, we could conclude that:

1. Chronic kidney disease patients on waiting list for renal transplantation present higher scores in the major dimensions of

quality of life, including functional capacity, physical functioning, pain, social life, emotional and mental health.

2. Patients present a major improvement in mental health, sleep quality, fatigue, physical and functional components of HRQoL after kidney transplantation.

3. Immunosuppressive treatment adverse effects might lead to deteriorated HRQoL in transplanted patients.

4. Anemia and lower urinary tract symptoms should be addressed properly in order to further improve HRQoL in transplanted patients.

5. Children rehabilitation after renal transplantation should focus on both physical activity and psychological state

6. Sexual dysfunction is less frequently observed in transplanted patients compared to those on dialysis.

7. Adherence to treatment and factors affecting external appearance should be carefully addressed in adolescent renal transplant patients.

Kidney transplantation represents the only definite known treatment of end stage renal disease. When carefully planned and performed it will lead to both improved survival and health related quality of life of patients with advanced chronic kidney disease.

ACKNOWLEDGEMENT

None Declared.

CONFLICT OF INTEREST

None Declared.

REFERENCES

Beck, A. T., Ward, C. H., Mendelson, M., Mock, J., & Erbaugh, J. (1961). An inventory for measuring depression. Arch Gen.Psychiatry, 4, 561-571.

Chien, C. H., Wang, H. H., Chiang, Y. J., Chu, S. H., Liu, H. E., & Liu, K. L. (2010). Quality of life after laparoscopic donor nephrectomy. Transplant.Proc., 42, 696-698.

Cornella, C., Brustia, M., Lazzarich, E., Cofano, F., Ceruso, A., Barbe, M. C., Fenoglio, R., Cella, D., & Stratta, P. (2008). Quality of life in renal transplant patients over 60 years of age. Transplant.Proc., 40, 1865-1866.

Dew, M. A., Switzer, G. E., Goycoolea, J. M., Allen, A. S., DiMartini, A., Kormos, R. L., & Griffith, B. P. (1997). Does transplantation produce quality of life benefits? A quantitative analysis of the literature. Transplantation, 64, 1261-1273.

Diseth, T. H., Tangeraas, T., Reinfjell, T., & Bjerre, A. (2011). Kidney transplantation in childhood: mental health and quality of life of children and caregivers. Pediatr.Nephrol., 26, 1881-1892.

Dobbels, F., Decorte, A., Roskams, A., & Van Damme-Lombaerts, R. (2010). Health-related quality of life, treatment adherence, symptom experience and depression in adolescent renal transplant patients. Pediatr.Transplant., 14, 216-223.

Falger, J., Landolt, M. A., Latal, B., Ruth, E. M., Neuhaus, T. J., & Laube, G. F. (2008). Outcome after renal transplantation. Part II: quality of life and psychosocial adjustment. Pediatr.Nephrol., 23, 1347-1354.

Franke, G. H., Trampenau, C., & Reimer, J. (2006). Switching from cyclosporine to tacrolimus leads to improved disease-specific quality of life in patients after kidney transplantation. Transplant.Proc., 38, 1293-1294.

Gentile, S., Jouve, E., Dussol, B., Moal, V., Berland, Y., & Sambuc, R. (2008). Development and validation of a French patient-based health-related quality of life instrument in kidney transplant: the ReTransQoL. Health Qual.Life Outcomes., 6, 78.

Gilson, B. S., Gilson, J. S., Bergner, M., Bobbit, R. A., Kressel, S., Pollard, W. E., & Vesselago, M. (1975). The sickness impact profile. Development of an outcome measure of health care. Am.J.Public Health, 65, 1304-1310.

Goldstein, S. L., Graham, N., Burwinkle, T., Warady, B., Farrah, R., & Varni, J. W. (2006). Health-related quality of life in pediatric patients with ESRD. Pediatr.Nephrol., 21, 846-850.

Griva, K., Davenport, A., Harrison, M., & Newman, S. P. (2012). The impact of treatment transitions between dialysis and transplantation on illness cognitions and quality of life - A prospective study. Br.J.Health Psychol., 17, 812-827.

Guleria, S., Reddy, V. S., Bora, G. S., Sagar, R., Bhowmik, D., & Mahajan, S. (2011). The quality of life of women volunteering as live-related kidney donors in India. Natl.Med.J.India, 24, 342-344.

Hays, R. D., Kallich, J. D., & Mapes, D. L. (1996). Kidney Disease Quality of Life Short Form (KDQOL-SF36) Version 1.3 A manual for use and scoring. Santa Monica.

Kalantar-Zadeh, K., Kopple, J. D., Deepak, S., Block, D., & Block, G. (2002). Food intake characteristics of hemodialysis patients as obtained by food frequency questionnaire. J.Ren Nutr., 12, 17-31.

Karam, V. H., Gasquet, I., Delvart, V., Hiesse, C., Dorent, R., Danet, C., Samuel, D., Charpentier, B., Gandjbakhch, I., Bismuth, H., & Castaing, D. (2003). Quality of life in adult survivors beyond 10 years after liver, kidney, and heart transplantation. Transplantation, 76, 1699-1704.

Kawada, N., Moriyama, T., Ichimaru, N., Imamura, R., Matsui, I., Takabatake, Y., Nagasawa, Y., Isaka, Y., Kojima, Y., Kokado, Y., Rakugi, H., Imai, E., & Takahara, S. (2009). Negative effects of anemia on quality of life and its improvement by complete correction of anemia by administration of recombinant human erythropoietin in posttransplant patients. Clin.Exp.Nephrol., 13, 355-360.

Kugler, C., Maeding, I., & Russell, C. L. (2011). Non-adherence in patients on chronic hemodialysis: an international comparison study. J.Nephrol., 24, 366-375.

Lam, L. W., Twinn, S. F., & Chan, S. W. (2010). Self-reported adherence to a therapeutic regimen among patients undergoing continuous ambulatory peritoneal dialysis. J.Adv.Nurs., 66, 763-773.

Mason, N. A. (2011). Polypharmacy and medication-related complications in the chronic kidney disease patient. Curr.Opin.Nephrol.Hypertens., 20, 492-497.

Minnee, R. C., Bemelman, W. A., Polle, S. W., van Koperen, P. J., Ter, M. S., Donselaar-van der Pant KA, Bemelman, F. J., & Idu, M. M. (2008). Older living kidney donors: surgical outcome and quality of life. Transplantation, 86, 251-256.

Mitsui, T., Shimoda, N., Morita, K., Tanaka, H., Moriya, K., & Nonomura, K. (2009). Lower urinary tract symptoms and their impact on quality of life after successful renal transplantation. Int.J.Urol., 16, 388-392.

Moloney, F. J., Keane, S., O'Kelly, P., Conlon, P. J., & Murphy, G. M. (2005). The impact of skin disease following renal transplantation on quality of life. Br.J.Dermatol., 153, 574-578.

Molzahn, A. E., Northcott, H. C., & Dossetor, J. B. (1997). Quality of life of individuals with end stage renal disease: perceptions of patients, nurses, and physicians. ANNA.J., 24, 325-333.

Morales, J. M., Varo, E., & Lazaro, P. (2012). Immunosuppressant treatment adherence, barriers to adherence and quality of life in renal and liver transplant recipients in Spain. Clin.Transplant., 26, 369-376.

Muehrer, R. J. & Becker, B. N. (2005). Life after transplantation: new transitions in quality of life and psychological distress. Semin.Dial., 18, 124-131.

Neri, L., Dukes, J., Brennan, D. C., Salvalaggio, P. R., Seelam, S., Desiraju, S., & Schnitzler, M. (2011). Impaired renal function is associated with worse self-reported outcomes after kidney transplantation. Qual.Life Res., 20, 1689-1698.

Prasad, G. V., Nash, M. M., Keough-Ryan, T., & Shapiro, R. J. (2010). A quality of life comparison in cyclosporine- and tacrolimus-treated renal transplant recipients across Canada. J.Nephrol., 23, 274-281.

Rodrigue, J. R., Mandelbrot, D. A., Hanto, D. W., Johnson, S. R., Karp, S. J., & Pavlakis, M. (2011). A cross-sectional study of fatigue and sleep quality before and after kidney transplantation. Clin.Transplant., 25, E13-E21.

Santos, P. R. (2011). Comparison of quality of life between hemodialysis patients waiting and not waiting for kidney transplant from a poor region of Brazil. J.Bras.Nefrol., 33, 166-172.

Suzuki, A., Kenmochi, T., Maruyama, M., Akutsu, N., Iwashita, C., Otsuki, K., Ito, T., Matsumoto, I., & Asano, T. (2012). Changes in quality of life in deceased *versus* living-donor kidney transplantations. Transplant.Proc., 44, 287-289.

Szeifert, L., Bragg-Gresham, J. L., Thumma, J., Gillespie, B. W., Mucsi, I., Robinson, B. M., Pisoni, R. L., Disney, A., Combe, C., & Port, F. K. (2012). Psychosocial variables are associated with being wait-listed, but not with receiving a kidney transplant in the Dialysis Outcomes and Practice Patterns Study (DOPPS). Nephrol.Dial.Transplant., 27, 2107-2113.

Tong, A., Tjaden, L., Howard, K., Wong, G., Morton, R., & Craig, J. C. (2011). Quality of life of adolescent kidney transplant recipients. J.Pediatr., 159, 670-675.

Toorians, A. W., Janssen, E., Laan, E., Gooren, L. J., Giltay, E. J., Oe, P. L., Donker, A. J., & Everaerd, W. (1997). Chronic renal failure and sexual functioning: clinical status *versus* objectively assessed sexual response. Nephrol.Dial.Transplant., 12, 2654-2663.

Tovazzi, M. E. & Mazzoni, V. (2012). Personal paths of fluid restriction in patients on hemodialysis. Nephrol.Nurs.J., 39, 207-215.

Wong, G., Howard, K., Chapman, J., Pollock, C., Chadban, S., Salkeld, G., Tong, A., Williams, N., Webster, A., & Craig, J. C. (2012). How do people with chronic kidney disease value cancer-related quality of life? Nephrology.(Carlton.), 17, 32-41.

CHAPTER 6

Influence of Kidney Transplantation on Cognitive Function in End - Stage Kidney Disease Patients

Josipa Radic[1,*], Mislav Radic[1] and Katarina Dodig Curkovic[2]

[1]Department of Internal Medicine, University Hospital Center Split, University of Split School of Medicine, Split, Croatia and [2]Department of Psychiatry, University Hospital Center Osijek, University of Osijek School of Medicine, Osijek, Croatia

Abstract: Kidney failure is believed to have a negative impact on cognitive function, and cognitive impairment is common in people with chronic kidney disease and end - stage kidney disease (ESKD). Diagnosis of cognitive impairment in this population of patients is important because cognitive impairment may have a role in the patient's understanding and acceptance of ESKD care, both at the initiation and duration of kidney replacement therapy. The pathophysiology of cognitive impairment is uncertain; it is a complex and probably multifactorial process. It is not known whether cognitive impairment is mediated by direct toxic effects of uraemia *per se*, or is attributed to a high prevalence of predisposing risk factors among ESKD patients and side effects of dialysis treatment. Recent studies noted that cognitive impairment in patients with end stage renal disease is likely to improve with successful kidney transplantation and that early beneficial effects of kidney transplantation on cognitive function are not transient and were still evident one year following successful kidney transplantation. On the other hand, some cognitive limitations may still be present in kidney transplant recipients and cognitive impairment in kidney transplant recipients may impact decision-making as well the ability to adhere to transplantation recommendations, such as dietary modification and complex medication compliance. Delay in diagnosis and treatment of cognitive impairment may result in medication non adherence and subsequent severe adverse effects such as acute graft rejection. Periodic assessment of end stage renal disease patient's cognitive function prior and post transplantation should be one of the parameters to be considered on evaluating outcomes after kidney transplantation.

Keywords: Cognitive function, kidney tran splantation, end - stage kidney disease, kidney failure, cognitive impairment, kidney replacement therapy, adherence, compliance, medical regimen, hemodialysis.

*****Address correspondence to Josipa Radic:** Department of Internal Medicine, University Hospital Center Split, University of Split School of Medicine, Split, Croatia; Tel: 00385915027100; Fax: 0038521557385; E-mail: jdodig@net.hr

Paraskevi Theofilou (Ed)

INTRODUCTION

Chronic kidney disease (CKD) is the permanent loss of kidney function and it is a rapidly growing global health problem with prevalence of 15% in developed nations (Fox *et al.*, 2006; Nitsch *et al.*, 2006). Given the pathogenic progression of kidney disease, patients with CKD are at high risk for progression to the end - stage kidney disease (ESKD) - a progressive, debilitating, chronic illness that requires nursing and medical interventions that include dialysis or kidney transplantation, education on lifestyle alterations, and dietary and fluid restrictions to maintain patients' long-term survival. The number of people known to have ESKD worldwide is growing rapidly as a result of improved diagnostic capabilities and also the global epidemic of type 2 diabetes, hypertension and other causes of chronic kidney disease.

With the increased incidence of ESKD worldwide due to an aging world population, and the increasing prevalence of comorbid diseases (Kurella, Covinsky, Collins, & Chertow, 2007; Lok, Oliver, Rothwell, & Hux, 2004), the demand for renal replacement therapy is also in rise. In ESKD, kidney function can be replaced by three main medical treatment modalities: hemodialysis (HD), peritoneal dialysis (PD) or by kidney transplantation. The best treatment for a patient who is very close to ESKD is pre-emptive transplantation, but transplantation generally does not happen because of an insufficient number of donors. Pre-emptive transplantation is an attractive option for patients because of reduced costs and improved graft survival (Meier-Kriesche, & Kaplan, 2002). Therefore, pre-emptive transplantation is associated with a 25% reduction in transplant failure and 16% reduction in mortality compared to recipients receiving a transplant after starting dialysis treatment (Kasiske *et al.*, 2002).

The two major dialysis types, HD and PD, are not only different from one another technically, but also with regard to the expectations of patients pertaining to the effort involved. Each dialysis type has its advantages and disadvantages and has a different level of impact on patients' physical, psychological and social health, and each places its own limitations on patients' lifestyle (Lindqvist, Carlsson, & Sjoden, 2000). HD or PD only partially correct the uremia and also render necessary substantial lifestyle changes. On the other hand, kidney transplantation is the treatment that most resembles normal kidney function and eliminates the limitations that dialysis causes in daily life.

COGNITIVE FUNCTION IN END STAGE RENAL DISEASE PATIENTS

ESKD can have an impact on patients' quality of life (QoL), potentially affecting their physical and mental health, functional status, independence, general well-being, personal relationships and social functioning. Awareness of patient satisfaction and QoL has been increasing and health-related QoL issues are now recognized as important outcome measures in health care, cost-effective analyses of the efficacy of medical care and clinical trials.

Kidney failure is believed to have a negative impact on cognitive function, and cognitive impairment is common in people with CKD (Elias *et al.*, 2009; Madan, Kalra, Agarwal, & Tandon, 2007) and ESRD (Murray *et al.*, 2006). People with CKD have lover cognitive scores and higher rate of cognitive decline than those without CKD (Buchman *et al.*, 2009; Khatri *et al.*, 2009). Cognitive impairment is associated with the severity of kidney disease, with impairment significantly more prevalent in dialysis patients than individuals with stage 3–4 chronic kidney disease (Kurella, Chertow, Luan, & Yaffe, 2004a; Madan *et al.*, 2007). Change in cognitive function may be a major determinant in patients' QoL. Moderate to severe cognitive impairment likely is undiagnosed, but highly prevalent in ESKD patients. (Kurella, Chertow, *et al.*, 2004; Pereira *et al.*, 2007; Sehgal, Grey, DeOreo, & Whitehouse, 1997).

Cognitive impairment in ESKD patients is an important question because cognitive impairment has been associated with decreased QoL in ESKD patients (Gokal, 1993) and may impact decision-making as well the ability to adhere to dialysis and transplantation recommendations, such as dietary modification and complex medication compliance. It has been demonstrated that cognitive impairment is an independent predictor of mortality in dialysis patients (Griva *et al.*, 2010).

Furthermore, diagnosis of cognitive impairment in dialysis population is important because cognitive impairment may have a role in the patient's understanding and acceptance of ESKD care, both at the initiation and duration of kidney replacement therapy (Pereira, Weiner, Scott, & Sarnak, 2005).

Prevalence of Cognitive Impairment in ESKD Patients

In study by Murray *et al.*, (Murray *et al.*, 2006) more than one-third (37%) of 338 hemodialysis patients were classified with severe cognitive impairment, 36.1% with moderate impairment, 13.9% with mild impairment, and 12.7% with normal cognition. It is important to note that only 2.9% had a documented history of cognitive impairment. Similar to HD patients, two-thirds of peritoneal dialysis patients had moderate to severe cognitive impairment (Kalirao *et al.*, 2011). The most frequently reported cognitive problems in dialysis population include memory deficits, reduced mental efficiency, decreased psychomotor speed, and impaired attention (Griva *et al.*, 2004; Griva *et al.*, 2010; Murray *et al.*, 2006).

Risk Factors for Cognitive Impairment in ESKD Patients

The pathophysiology of cognitive impairment is uncertain; it is a complex and probably multifactorial process. It is not known whether cognitive impairment is mediated by direct toxic effects of uremia *per se*, or is attributed to a high prevalence of predisposing risk factors among ESKD patients and side effects of dialysis treatment (Table 1). It is well known that dialysis patients have a high prevalence of both cognitive impairment and brain abnormalities (Fazekas *et al.*, 1995; Murray *et al.*, 2006; Sehgal *et al.*, 1997). The structural brain abnormalities include cerebral atrophy, white matter hyperintensities, silent brain infarcts and leucoaraiosis (Fazekas *et al.*, 1995; Geissler *et al.*, 1995; Sehgal *et al.*, 1997). White matter lesions have been independently associated with severity of kidney disease (Ikram *et al.*, 2008).

Table 1: Risk Factors that may be related to Cognitive Impairment in Dialysis Patients.

Hemodialysis procedure	Hemodialysis related hypotension
	Thrombotic events during hemodialysis
	Cerebral hypoperfusion
	Cerebral edema (dialysis disequilibrium syndrome)
	Hyperviscosity of the blood (hemoconcentration)
	Dialysis dose

Table 1: contd...

Cerebrovascular disease	Cerebral brain atrophy
	Silent lacunars infarction
	White matter hyperintensities
	Leukoaraiosis
	Stroke
	Atherosclerosis
Vascular risk factors	Hypertension
	Diabetes
	Hypercholesterolemia
	Hemostatic abnormalities
	Hypercoaguable states
	Inflammation
	Oxidative stress
Nonvascular risk factors	Age
	Smoking
	Education
	Anemia
	Hyperparathyroidism
	Depression
	Malnutrition
	Sleep disturbances
	Polypharmacy (retention of medication metabolites)
Cardiovascular disease	Myocardial infarction
	Atrial fibrillation
Others	Uremic solutes Parathyroid hormone

Dialysis Dose and Cognitive Function

In the current era of increased dialysis dose, cognitive impairment is still an important and highly prevalent, and underdiagnosed problem in ESKD population (Giang *et al.*, 2011; Kurella, Luan, Yaffe, & Chertow, 2004; Murray *et al.*, 2006). Older studies have suggested that decreased dialysis dose may be associated with worse cognitive function in hemodialysis patients (Hart, Pederson, Czerwinski, & Adams, 1983; Umans, & Pliskin, 1998). In contrast to previous studies, equilibrated Kt/V≥1.2 was associated with severe cognitive impairment in the study of the prevalence of cognitive impairment in 338 HD patients (Murray *et al.*, 2006). Association between high dialysis dose and severe cognitive impairment is unexpected and not well explained. It is important to note that in the current era of increased dialysis dose Giang at al. (Giang *et al.*, 2011) have not demonstrated any association between higher dialysis dose and better performance on any measure of cognitive testing. The persistence of cognitive impairment despite clinically adequate dialysis dose delivery indicates that other factors also contribute to the brain dysfunction (Marsh *et al.*, 1991).

The Hemodialysis Process and Cognitive Function

A few recent studies suggested that the decline in cognitive function can be halted and reversed after successful kidney transplantation (Griva *et al.*, 2006; Harciarek, Biedunkiewicz, Lichodziejewska-Niemierko, Debska-Slizien, & Rutkowski, 2011; Radic, Ljutic, Radic, Kovacic, Dodig-Curkovic, *et al.*, 2011a), suggesting a major rule of the uremia or the HD process itself in cognitive impairment. However, the persistence of neurobehavioral impairment despite clinically adequate HD indicates that other factors also contribute to the brain dysfunction (Marsh *et al.*, 1991). Because the prevalence of cognitive impairment observed among maintenance HD patients was far greater than previously observed in patients with earlier stages of CKD the investigators hypothesized that that the HD process itself may directly contribute to the development of cognitive impairment, possibly by inducing cerebral ischemia or cerebral edema through intravascular volume loss and fluid shift during HD session (Griva *et al.*, 2003; Murray *et al.*, 2007). Global cognitive function varies significantly during HD cycle, being worst during HD and best shortly before the session or the day after. An acute decrease in cognitive function during HD across multiple cognitive spheres, including attention, executive function, and memory was found (Murray *et al.*, 2007). Those results suggest that the worst time to communicate with HD patients appears to be during the HD session.

Dialysis Modality and Cognitive Function

While it is sufficiently well documented that ESKD has been linked with change in cognitive function, little is known about influence of different dialysis modalities on cognitive function. The effect of dialysis modality on risk of cognitive impairment is unclear. Although a considerable number of articles on ESKD have been published, there are a limited number of studies comparing cognitive function in HD and CAPD patients. Some data from older studies data suggest that patients with ESKD treated with PD had consistently better cognitive function than patients treated with HD (Buoncristiani *et al.*, 1993; Tilki, Akpolat, Tunali, Kara, & Onar, 2004; Wolcott *et al.*, 1988). These results may not reflect the dialysis procedure itself but selection bias as to who is receiving which modality of dialysis treatment. A selected group of dialysis patients was not matched for important demographic variables, including age or level of education. The differences in cognitive functions between the two dialysis modalities could also be due to differences in cognitive functions prior to the start of dialysis, which makes a comparison between the modalities difficult. Some authors concluded that the previously observed apparent difference between two modalities of dialysis treatments resulted either from very low dialysis delivery or comparison with poorly matched controls (Radic *et al.*, 2010). Also, in a recent study they have demonstrated that well-dialyzed, well-nourished and medically stable HD patients had no cognitive dysfunction in comparison with well-dialyzed, well-nourished, medically stable and demographically matched PD patients (Radic, Ljutic, Radic, Kovacic, Sain, *et al.*, 2011b).

COGNITIVE FUNCTION IN KIDNEY TRANSPLANTANT RECIPIENTS

Definition and Outcome of Kidney Transplantation

Kidney transplantation is replacement of nonworking kidneys with a healthy kidney from another person (the donor). Therefore, kidney transplantation is the treatment of choice and should be strongly considered for all patients with ESKD who are medically suitable (Suthanthiran, & Strom, 1994). A successful kidney transplant offers enhanced quality and duration of life and is more effective (medically and economically) than any modality of long-term dialysis therapy (Tonelli *et al.*, 2011). In the last 20 years, better understanding of the benefits of combined immunosuppressant drugs coupled with improved organ matching and preservation, as well as chemoprophylaxis of opportunistic infections, have all contributed to a progressive improvement in clinical outcomes.

During the past decade, there has been significant improvement in graft and patient survival, mostly attributed to better immunosuppressive drugs, improvements in surgical techniques and postoperative care, as well as early diagnosis and treatment of acute rejection, and bacterial and viral infection episodes. In parallel to better patient care and new immunosuppressive therapies the median survival of renal allograft improved continuously (Hariharan *et al.*, 2000). Data from the Organ Procurement and Transplantation Network for transplants performed in 2002-2004 show that the 1-year survival rate for grafts from living donors is approximately 96.4 % and the rate for deceased donor grafts is approximately 92.1% (Bajwa *et al.*, 2007).

The major goal of successful kidney transplantation is the achievement of maximal quality and quantity of life while minimizing the effects of disease, prolong survival and also the costs of care for dialysis patients. Studies on outcome after kidney transplantation have traditionally measured post-operative survival and complication rates. Advances in kidney transplant procedures and immunosuppressive therapies have increased dramatically over the last decades. The introduction of cyclosporine as immunosuppressive drug in the mid-1980s was a major advance.

Hand in hand with all these achievements, greater attention has been given to long term quality of life in this population of patients. Successful kidney transplantation is associated with improvement in depression, IQ and life satisfaction (Kurella, Luan, *et al.*, 2004). Although a successful transplantation results in restored health and quality of life (Gritsch, 1996; Laupacis *et al.*, 1996; Ponton *et al.*, 2001), the influence of successful kidney transplantation on cognitive function is still not well understood. Evidence suggests that cognitive function significantly improves following successful kidney transplantation. Kidney transplant recipients showed better cognitive function measured by various neuropsychological tests, compared with ESKD patients treated with various dialysis methods.

There are many reasons for the improvement in the cognitive function after successful kidney transplantation and they may all occur simultaneously. Fluid intake and diet restriction are raised. Many substances come to normal levels after kidney transplantation but the link between biochemical markers of kidney function and cognitive performance in kidney transplant recipients were weak and inconsistent.

Beneficial Effect of Kidney Transplantation on Cognitive Function

Although a considerable number of articles on cognitive impairment in patients with ESKD have been published, there are a limited number of studies comparing cognitive function in dialysis population before and after successful kidney transplantation. The current literature on the cognitive functioning after successful kidney transplantation is based predominantly on cross-sectional study or prospective studies that assessed small samples with brief neuropsychological assessments. Recent studies noted that cognitive impairment in patients with ESKD is likely to improve with successful kidney transplantation (Gritsch, 1996; Laupacis *et al.*, 1996; Ponton *et al.*, 2001). Most of these studies suggest that significant pre- to post transplantation improvements occur only in certain neuropsychological tests and not across all the cognitive domains assessed. In an old study Teschan at al. (Teschan, Ginn, Bourne, & Ward, 1976) studied eight repeatedly during HD treatment and 4-23 months after successful kidney transplantation using electroencephalograms (EEG) and neuropsychological tests of attention and memory. They found a significant improvement in the EEG, choice reaction times and memory tests scores following transplantation.

The one area where clear evidence of cognitive improvement following transplantation was found in previous study is memory. There were no statistically significant improvements in measures of attention, visual planning, mental processing speed and motor abilities six months after successful kidney transplantation (Griva *et al.*, 2006). It may be that the memory tests used in this study are more stringent and sensitive than those tests used to assess attention and concentration and motor abilities. One previous study compared cognitive functioning between dialysis and transplanted patients using neuropsychological tests that assess learning and verbal recall, attention and concentration and psychomotor speed. Transplanted patients performed significantly better than dialysis patients on the two memory tasks and two out of the four tests of attention. No differences were found in the motor task. Therefore, their results revealed that neuropsychological advantage of transplantation relative to dialysis is evident mainly in verbal memory. This finding contrasts with commonly held views that successful kidney transplantation should result in amelioration of cognitive functioning. Authors concluded that these findings might be related to the characteristics of the dialysis sample, which consisted of clinically stabile and adequately dialyzed patients or to technological improvements of dialysis procedure over recent years (Griva *et al.*, 2004). Kramer *et al.,* (Kramer *et al.*, 1996) found that P300 event-related potential latency decreased (improved) and P300 amplitude increased (improved), indicating significant mental improvement following transplantation. Psychometric tests (Trail making test and Mini-mental state) tend to improve, indicating improved psychomotor performance following transplantation, but psychometric improvements did not yield statistical significance probably due to a lower sensitivity compared to P300 (Grimm *et al.*, 1990).

Also, most of the previous studies have suffered from a lack of standardization of dialysis adequacy, well matched controls groups, insufficient neuropsychological tests, and performed cross-sectional comparison, which made the interpretation of their otherwise promising findings somewhat limited. In contrast, two recent studies showed that successful kidney transplantation leads to significant improvement in performance on the test of motor/psychomotor speed, visual planning, memory, and abstract thinking (Harciarek, Biedunkiewicz, Lichodziejewska-Niemierko, Debska-Slizien, & Rutkowski, 2009; Harciarek *et al.*, 2011).

Long-lasting Effects of Successful Kidney Transplantation on Cognitive Function

Some authors suggested that early beneficial effects of kidney transplantation on cognitive function are not transient and were still evident one year following successful kidney transplantation (Harciarek *et al.*, 2011) and cognitive performance might even be improved in longer time following transplantation (Griva *et al.*, 2006). Further improvement in cognitive function might be expected at longer post transplantation follow-up as patients continue to recover both medically and functionally and are put on lower dosage of immunosuppressive medication.

The results from a recent study have shown significantly better performance on cognitive and psychomotor tests that assess processing speed, attention, short time memory, convergent thinking and executive functioning 20.5 ± 8.5 months after successful kidney transplantation. It is important to note that neuropsychological measures used in this study did assess cognitive and psychomotor domains found to be particularly impaired in ESKD patients on maintenance HD such as memory, mental efficiency, psychomotor speed, attention, and executive function (Gelb, Shapiro, Hill, & Thornton, 2008; Griva *et al.*, 2010; Murray *et al.*, 2006; Pereira *et al.*, 2007). These findings of improved cognitive function in adequately dialyzed patients (Kt/V≥ 1.2) after successful kidney transplantation suggest that kidney transplantation is superior to adequate HD in improving cognitive function in HD patients.

In these studies each research team took a different approach and used different neuropsychological instruments to test cognitive performance in ESKD patients prior and post- transplantation which makes comparison of all results difficult (Table **2**).

Table 2: Cognitive Function assessed and associated Neuropsychological Test used in Kidney Transplantant Recipients.

TEST	COGNITIVE FUNCTION ASSESSED
California Verbal Learning Test-Second Edition (CVLT-II)	verbal learning and memory
Trail Making Test Forms A and B (TMT)	attention, visual scanning, motor speed and planning ability
Colour-Word Interference Test	executive functioning (verbal inhibition of a dominant response)
Symbol Digit Modalities Test (SDMT)	visual attention - concentration, oculomotor abilities, hand-eye coordination
Rey Auditory Verbal Learning Test (RAVLT)	immediate memory, retrieval from verbal short-term memory storage
Grooved Pegboard (GP)	fine motor co-ordination and manual dexterity
Complex Reactionmeter Drenovac (CRD series)	perceptive abilities, memory, thinking, psychomotor reactions, attention and functional disturbances
Benton Visual Retention Test (BVRT)	visual perception, visual memory, visuoconstructive abilities

Table 2: contd…

Brief Visual Memory Test – Revised (BVMT-R)	visual learning
Rey-Osterrieth Complex Figure test (RCF)	visual-spatial memory, construction, organization ability
Digit span subtest of the Polish adaption of the Wechsler Adult Intelligence Scale – Revised (WAIS-R-PL)	attention and working memory
Finger Tapping Test	motor abilities
Mini-Mental State Examination (MMSE)	general cognitive status, screening test for cognitive impairment
Polish adaptation of Zigmond and Snaith's Hospital Anxiety and Depression Scale (HAD)	depression and anxiety
Center for Epidemiological Studies-Depression Scale (CES-D)	depression

Cognitive Impairment and Non adherence to Prescribed Medical Regimens in Kidney Transplant Recipients

Kidney transplantation is a chronic illness, in which transplant patients are bound to life-long medical follow-up and drug treatment. Cognitive deficits such are memory and executive functioning difficulties may be present following successful kidney transplantation. Given the fact that reduced cognitive performance has been identified in kidney transplant recipients, it will be paramount to elucidate the consequences in terms of medication adherence, ability to return to work and other functional outcomes (Gelb *et al.*, 2008).

All patients should have a pretransplant psychosocial evaluation by experienced competent individual to assess for cognitive impairment, mental illness, nonadherence to therapy and drug or alcohol abuse (Knoll *et al.*, 2005). Cognitive impairment in kidney transplant recipients may impact decision-making as well the ability to adhere to transplantation recommendations, such as dietary modification and complex medication compliance. Patient nonadherence to therapy is a contraindication to kidney transplantation. Kidney transplantation should be delayed until patients have demonstrated adherence for at least 6 months (Knoll *et al.*, 2005).

Nonadherence of transplant recipients to prescribed medical regimens has been identified as a major risk factor for rejection and allograft loss (Denhaerynck *et al.*, 2005; Pinsky *et al.*, 2009). In clinical trials, nonadherence rates as high as 43 to 78% have been reported (Claxton, Cramer, & Pierce, 2001; Cramer *et al.*, 2003). Older patients may have lower verbal memory skills and cognitive impairment that may affect compliance. Some authors found better verbal memory to be independently associated with the use of medication schedules and that better executive functioning was strongly associated with adherence to prescription instructions in elderly patients (Stoehr *et al.*, 2008). As a threat to optimal outcomes after kidney transplantation, cognitive impairment and nonadherence to prescribed medical regimens are worthy of attention and intervention. Successful intervention to improve cognitive function and adherence must be multidimensional.

Immunosuppressive Medication and Cognitive Function in Kidney Transplant Recipients

Cognitive limitations may still be present in kidney transplant recipients and the failure of kidney transplant to fully reverse cognitive problems associated with ESKD and/or dialysis could have been a result of early adverse effects of high doses of immunosuppressive therapy (Gelb *et al.*, 2008). Some kidney transplant patients show cognitive, emotional, and behavioral changes as part of possible neurotoxic effects associated with immunosuppressive medication, especially tacrolimus. The recent study evaluated effects of immunosuppressive drugs on cognitive tasks. Patients treated with sirolimus and cyclosporine reported some of the noncognitive side effects related to immunosuppressive treatment. Attention and working memory impairment were observed in patients treated with sirolimus or tacrolimus. Performance of cyclosporine-treated subjects was similar to that of healthy volunteer controls. Since the mood, anxiety, and sleep patterns measured were unaffected, authors concluded that the cognitive deficit found was partly related to treatment (Martinez-Sanchis *et al.*, 2011). In other study neuropsychological tests score were found to be equivalent in patients on cyclosporine and those on tacrolimus (Griva *et al.*, 2004).

Anemia and Cognitive Function in Kidney Transplant

It is well known that anemia is a frequent complication of ESKD. Inadequate production of erythropoietin by the failing kidneys leads to decreased stimulation of the bone marrow to produce red blood cells. Anemia of ESKD develops early and worsens with progressive renal insufficiency. As the diseased kidney loses its ability to produce the erythropoietin essential to the production of hemoglobin, anemia ensues. In patients on dialysis, untreated anemia can result in objective cognitive deficits (Nissenson, 1992) and anemia has been identified as a risk factor for cognitive impairment in HD patients.

In modern renal replacement treatment, recombinant erythropoietin (rHuEPO) is an unavoidable drug for correcting anemia in patients with ESKD. Furthermore, correction of anemia with rHuEPO treatment has been shown to improve the measure of cognition (Singh *et al.*, 2006) and social functioning (Moreno, Sanz-Guajardo, Lopez-Gomez, Jofre, & Valderrabano, 2000). It still remains unknown whether this is solely due to an improvement in the blood count or an independent effect of supplementation with rHuEPO (Cerami, Brines, Ghezzi, Cerami, & Itri, 2002). On the other hand, a recent study discovered that the physiological effects of rHuEPO go far beyond erythropoiesis. High expression of EPO and its receptor in the brain during embryonic development has led to the investigation of not only the neurotrophic role of EPO but also its neuroprotective properties. Recently, rHuEPO has received attention for neurobiological actions mediated through non-hematopoietic rHuEPO receptors in central nervous system (Brines & Cerami, 2005). Therefore, systemically administered EPO crosses the blood-brain barrier and has neuroprotective and neurotrophic effects in variety of different causes of brain injury (Gunnarson *et al.*, 2009).

Following successful kidney transplantation, with the rise in endogenous erythropoietin production, hemoglobin levels generally rise and normalize within the first two to 4 months (Kessler, 1995). There is a positive correlation between hemoglobin level and creatinine clearance in renal transplant patients (Nankivell, Allen, Oconnell, & Chapman, 1995; Qunibi *et al.*, 1991) probably a function of endogenous erythropoietin production by the graft (Besarab, Caro, Jarrell, Francos, & Erslev, 1987). An improvement in cognitive function has been described with kidney transplantation that is superior to that observed with correction of anemia with rHuEPO. Two recent prospective studies clearly demonstrated that beneficial and relatively long-lasting cognitive effects of a successful kidney transplantation that cannot be attributed to change in level of hemoglobin prior or post-transplantation, or learning effects of repeated administration of cognitive task (Harciarek *et al.*, 2011; Radic, Ljutic, Radic, Kovacic, Dodig-Curkovic, *et al.*, 2011).

Patophysiologically, increase in hemoglobin level to normal or near normal values with subsequent increase of cerebral oxygen delivery may account for the beneficial cerebral effects of successful kidney transplantation. Therefore, correction of anemia in kidney transplant recipients leads to disappearance of symptom such as fatigue, sleep and appetite disorders. Fluid intake and diet intake are raised. All those changes may lead to the improvement of nutritional status after kidney transplantation. Malnutrition is considered to be one of the late complications of chronic renal failure. It is frequent, affects quality of life, and is linked to increased risk of morbidity and mortality (Kalantar-Zadeh, Kopple, Block, & Humphreys, 2001). Many studies have reported the presence of malnutrition in a large number of dialysis patients (Aparicio *et al.*, 1999) and that malnutrition is related to cognitive performance in HD patients (Radic, Ljutic, Radic, Kovacic, Curkovic, *et al.*, 2011). Improvement in nutritional status after kidney transplantation may be related to improvement in cognitive performance.

CONCLUDING REMARKS

Successful kidney transplantation was recently shown to lead to improvement in cognitive function of ESKD patients. The early beneficial effects of transplantation are not transient and cognitive performance might be even improved in time following successful kidney transplantation. Although no longer dependant on dialysis to survive, kidney transplant patients continue to have a numerous of medical problems and require numerous medications, including immunosuppressive drugs, antihypertensive, antibiotics, and antiviral agents.

Cognitive limitations may still be present in kidney transplant recipients. Therefore, kidney transplant recipients are at risk for cognitive impairment because of complex medical conditions that require frequent tests and follow-ups, new immunosuppressive medications such as corticosteroids, and the significant impact on lifestyle and work status, especially in the early phase of their transplantation. Delay in diagnosis and treatment of cognitive impairment may result in medication nonadherence and subsequent severe adverse effects such as acute graft rejection.

Cognitive impairment in ESKD patients prior and post-transplantation is important area of health and is not covered in the guidelines, and there are limitations because there is an overall lack of studies and research in this aspect of care despite its importance. Future studies are needed to determine the optimal approach to screening and managing cognitive deficits in ESKD patients prior and post kidney transplantation.

All practitioners caring for ESKD patients need to be aware of cognitive impairment, particularly when instructing patients and family members in patient care. As ESKD population grows older and treatment and prognosis of patients with ESKD and kidney transplant recipients improve, the prevention, recognition, and treatment of cognitive impairment will be of major importance. Periodic assessment of an ERKD patient's cognitive function should be one of the basic parameters to be considered on evaluating outcomes after kidney transplantation. Also, the prospective, multicenter studies with larger cohort are required to better understand the complexity of cognitive function recovery after successful kidney transplantation and to determine the potential modifiers of such recovery.

ACKNOWLEDGEMENT

None Declared.

CONFLICT OF INTEREST

None Declared.

REFERENCES

Aparicio, M., Cano, N., Chauveau, P., Azar, R., Canaud, B., Flory, A.,Leverve, X. (1999). Nutritional status of haemodialysis patients: a French national cooperative study. French Study Group for Nutrition in Dialysis. *Nephrol Dial Transplant, 14*(7), 1679-1686.

Bajwa, M., Cho, Y. W., Pham, P. T., Shah, T., Danovitch, G., Wilkinson, A., & Bunnapradist, S. (2007). Donor biopsy and kidney transplant outcomes: an analysis using the Organ Procurement and Transplantation Network/United Network for Organ Sharing (OPTN/UNOS) database. *Transplantation, 84*(11), 1399-1405.

Besarab, A., Caro, J., Jarrell, B. E., Francos, G., & Erslev, A. J. (1987). Dynamics of Erythropoiesis Following Renal-Transplantation. *Kidney International, 32*(4), 526-536.

Brines, M., & Cerami, A. (2005). Emerging biological roles for erythropoietin in the nervous system. *Nat Rev Neurosci, 6*(6), 484-494. doi: 10.1038/nrn1687

Buchman, A. S., Tanne, D., Boyle, P. A., Shah, R. C., Leurgans, S. E., & Bennett, D. A. (2009). Kidney function is associated with the rate of cognitive decline in the elderly. *Neurology, 73*(12), 920-927.

Buoncristiani, U., Alberti, A., Gubbiotti, G., Mazzotta, G., Gallai, V., Quintaliani, G., & Gaburri, M. (1993). Better preservation of cognitive faculty in continuous ambulatory peritoneal dialysis. *Perit Dial Int, 13 Suppl 2*, S202-205.

Cerami, A., Brines, M., Ghezzi, P., Cerami, C., & Itri, L. M. (2002). Neuroprotective properties of epoetin alfa. [Review]. *Nephrol Dial Transplant, 17 Suppl 1*, 8-12.

Claxton, A. J., Cramer, J., & Pierce, C. (2001). A systematic review of the associations between dose regimens and medication compliance. *Clinical Therapeutics, 23*(8), 1296-1310.

Cramer, J., Rosenheck, R., Kirk, G., Krol, W., Krystal, J., & 425, V. N. S. G. (2003). Medication compliance feedback and monitoring in a clinical trial: Predictors and outcomes. *Value in Health, 6*(5), 566-573.

Denhaerynck, K., Dobbels, F., Cleemput, I., Desmyttere, A., Schafer-Keller, P., Schaub, S., & De Geest, S. (2005). Prevalence, consequences, and determinants of nonadherence in adult renal transplant patients: a literature review. *Transplant International, 18*(10), 1121-1133.

Elias, M. F., Elias, P. K., Seliger, S. L., Narsipur, S. S., Dore, G. A., & Robbins, M. A. (2009). Chronic kidney disease, creatinine and cognitive functioning. *Nephrol Dial Transplant, 24*(8), 2446-2452.

Fazekas, G., Fazekas, F., Schmidt, R., Kapeller, P., Offenbacher, H., & Krejs, G. J. (1995). Brain Mri Findings and Cognitive Impairment in Patients Undergoing Chronic-Hemodialysis Treatment. *Journal of the Neurological Sciences, 134*(1-2), 83-88.

Fox, C. S., Larson, M. G., Vasan, R. S., Guo, C. Y., Parise, H., Levy, D., Benjamin, E. J. (2006). Cross-sectional association of kidney function with valvular and annular calcification: the Framingham heart study. *J Am Soc Nephrol, 17*(2), 521-527.

Geissler, A., Frund, R., Kohler, S., Eichhorn, H. M., Kramer, B. K., & Feuerbach, S. (1995). Cerebral Metabolite Patterns in Dialysis Patients - Evaluation with H-1 Mr Spectroscopy. *Radiology, 194*(3), 693-697.

Gelb, S., Shapiro, R. J., Hill, A., & Thornton, W. L. (2008). Cognitive outcome following kidney transplantation. *Nephrol Dial Transplant, 23*(3), 1032-1038.

Giang, L. M., Weiner, D. E., Agganis, B. T., Scott, T., Sorensen, E. P., Tighiouart, H., & Sarnak, M. J. (2011). Cognitive Function and Dialysis Adequacy: No Clear Relationship. *Am J Nephrol, 33*(1), 33-38.

Gokal, R. (1993). Quality-of-Life in Patients Undergoing Renal Replacement Therapy. *Kidney International, 43*, S23-S27.

Grimm, G., Stockenhuber, F., Schneeweiss, B., Madl, C., Zeitlhofer, J., & Schneider, B. (1990). Improvement of Brain-Function in Hemodialysis-Patients Treated with Erythropoietin. *Kidney International, 38*(3), 480-486.

Gritsch, H. A. (1996). Renal transplantation - Improving the quality of life. *Journal of Urology, 156*(3), 889-889.

Griva, K., Hansraj, S., Thompson, D., Jayasena, D., Davenport, A., Harrison, M., & Newman, S. P. (2004). Neuropsychological performance after kidney transplantation: a comparison between transplant types and in relation to dialysis and normative data. *Nephrology Dialysis Transplantation, 19*(7), 1866-1874.

Griva, K., Newman, S. P., Harrison, M. J., Hankins, M., Davenport, A., Hansraj, S., & Thompson, D. (2003). Acute neuropsychological changes in hemodialysis and peritoneal dialysis patients. *Health Psychol, 22*(6), 570-578.

Griva, K., Stygall, J., Hankins, M., Davenport, A., Harrison, M., & Newman, S. P. (2010). Cognitive Impairment and 7-Year Mortality in Dialysis Patients. *American Journal of Kidney Diseases, 56*(4), 693-703.

Griva, K., Thompson, D., Jayasena, D., Davenport, A., Harrison, M., & Newman, S. P. (2006). Cognitive functioning pre- to post-kidney transplantation--a prospective study. *Nephrol Dial Transplant, 21*(11), 3275-3282.

Gunnarson, E., Song, Y. T., Kowalewski, J. M., Brismar, H., Brines, M., Cerami, A., Aperia, A. (2009). Erythropoietin modulation of astrocyte water permeability as a component of neuroprotection. *Proceedings of the National Academy of Sciences of the United States of America, 106*(5), 1602-1607.

Harciarek, M., Biedunkiewicz, B., Lichodziejewska-Niemierko, M., Debska-Slizien, A., & Rutkowski, B. (2009). Cognitive performance before and after kidney transplantation: A prospective controlled study of adequately dialyzed patients with end-stage renal disease. *Journal of the International Neuropsychological Society, 15*(5), 684-694.

Harciarek, M., Biedunkiewicz, B., Lichodziejewska-Niemierko, M., Debska-Slizien, A., & Rutkowski, B. (2011). Continuous cognitive improvement 1 year following successful kidney transplant. *Kidney International, 79*(12), 1353-1360.

Hariharan, S., Johnson, C. P., Bresnahan, B. A., Taranto, S. E., McIntosh, M. J., & Stablein, D. (2000). Improved graft survival after renal transplantation in the United States, 1988 to 1996. *N Engl J Med, 342*(9), 605-612.

Hart, R. P., Pederson, J. A., Czerwinski, A. W., & Adams, R. L. (1983). Chronic-Renal-Failure, Dialysis, and Neuropsychological Function. *Journal of Clinical Neuropsychology, 5*(4), 301-312.

Ikram, M. A., Vernooij, M. W., Hofman, A., Niessen, W. J., van der Lugt, A., & Breteler, M. M. B. (2008). Kidney function is related to cerebral small vessel disease. *Stroke, 39*(1), 55-61.

Kalantar-Zadeh, K., Kopple, J. D., Block, G., & Humphreys, M. H. (2001). A malnutrition-inflammation score is correlated with morbidity and mortality in maintenance hemodialysis patients. *American Journal of Kidney Diseases, 38*(6), 1251-1263.

Kalirao, P., Pederson, S., Foley, R. N., Kolste, A., Tupper, D., Zaun, D., Murray, A. M. (2011). Cognitive Impairment in Peritoneal Dialysis Patients. *American Journal of Kidney Diseases, 57*(4), 612-620.

Kasiske, B. L., Snyder, J. J., Matas, A. J., Ellison, M. D., Gill, J. S., & Kausz, A. T. (2002). Preemptive kidney transplantation: The advantage and the advantaged. *Journal of the American Society of Nephrology, 13*(5).

Kessler, M. (1995). Erythropoietin and Erythropoiesis in Renal-Transplantation. *Nephrology Dialysis Transplantation, 10*, 114-116.

Khatri, M., Nickolas, T., Moon, Y. P., Paik, M. C., Rundek, T., Elkind, M. S. V., Wright, C. B. (2009). CKD Associates with Cognitive Decline. *Journal of the American Society of Nephrology, 20*(11), 2427-2432.

Knoll, G., Cockfield, S., Blydt-Hansen, T., Baran, D., Kiberd, B., Landsberg, D., Cana, K. T. W. G. (2005). Canadian Society of Transplantation consensus guidelines on eligibility for kidney transplantation. *Canadian Medical Association Journal, 173*(10), 1181-1184.

Kramer, L., Madl, C., Stockenhuber, F., Yeganehfar, W., Eisenhuber, E., Derfler, K., Grimm, G. (1996). Beneficial effect of renal transplantation on cognitive brain function. *Kidney International, 49*(3), 833-838.

Kurella, M., Chertow, G. M., Luan, J., & Yaffe, K. (2004). Cognitive impairment in chronic kidney disease. *J Am Geriatr Soc, 52*(11), 1863-1869.

Kurella, M., Covinsky, K. E., Collins, A. J., & Chertow, G. M. (2007). Octogenarians and nonagenarians starting dialysis in the United States. *Ann Intern Med, 146*(3), 177-183.

Kurella, M., Luan, J., Yaffe, K., & Chertow, G. M. (2004a). Validation of the kidney disease quality of life (KDQOL) cognitive function subscale. *Kidney International, 66*(6), 2361-2367.

Laupacis, A., Keown, P., Pus, N., Krueger, H., Ferguson, B., Wong, C., & Muirhead, N. (1996). A study of the quality of life and cost-utility of renal transplantation. *Kidney International, 50*(1), 235-242.

Lindqvist, R., Carlsson, M., & Sjoden, P. O. (2000). Coping strategies and health-related quality of life among spouses of continuous ambulatory peritoneal dialysis, haemodialysis, and transplant patients. *Journal of Advanced Nursing, 31*(6), 1398-1408.

Lok, C. E., Oliver, M. J., Rothwell, D. M., & Hux, J. E. (2004). The growing volume of diabetes-related dialysis: a population based study. [Comparative Study]. *Nephrol Dial Transplant, 19*(12), 3098-3103.

Madan, P., Kalra, O. P., Agarwal, S., & Tandon, O. P. (2007). Cognitive impairment in chronic kidney disease. *Nephrol Dial Transplant, 22*(2), 440-444.

Marsh, J. T., Brown, W. S., Wolcott, D., Carr, C. R., Harper, R., Schweitzer, S. V., & Nissenson, A. R. (1991). Rhuepo Treatment Improves Brain and Cognitive Function of Anemic Dialysis Patients. *Kidney International, 39*(1), 155-163.

Martinez-Sanchis, S., Bernal, M. C., Montagud, J. V., Candela, G., Crespo, J., Sancho, A., & Pallardo, L. M. (2011). Effects of immunosuppressive drugs on the cognitive functioning of renal transplant recipients: A pilot study. *Journal of Clinical and Experimental Neuropsychology, 33*(9), 1016-1024.

Meier-Kriesche, H. U., & Kaplan, B. (2002). Waiting time on dialysis as the strongest modifiable risk factor for renal transplant outcomes - A paired donor kidney analysis. *Transplantation, 74*(10), 1377-1381.

Moreno, F., Sanz-Guajardo, D., Lopez-Gomez, J. M., Jofre, R., & Valderrabano, F. (2000). Increasing the hematocrit has a beneficial effect on quality of life and is safe in selected hemodialysis patients. Spanish Cooperative Renal Patients Quality of Life Study Group of the Spanish Society of Nephrology. *J Am Soc Nephrol, 11*(2), 335-342.

Murray, A. M., Pederson, S. L., Tupper, D. E., Hochhalter, A. K., Miller, W. A., Li, Q.,Foley, R. N. (2007). Acute variation in cognitive function in hemodialysis patients: a cohort study with repeated measures. *Am J Kidney Dis, 50*(2), 270-278.

Murray, A. M., Tupper, D. E., Knopman, D. S., Gilbertson, D. T., Pederson, S. L., Li, S., Kane, R. L. (2006). Cognitive impairment in hemodialysis patients is common. *Neurology, 67*(2), 216-223.

Nankivell, B. J., Allen, R. D. M., Oconnell, P. J., & Chapman, J. R. (1995). Erythrocytosis after Renal-Transplantation - Risk-Factors and Relationship with Gfr. *Clinical Transplantation, 9*(5), 375-382.

Nissenson, A. R. (1992). Epoetin and Cognitive Function. *American Journal of Kidney Diseases, 20*(1), 21-24.

Nitsch, D., Felber Dietrich, D., von Eckardstein, A., Gaspoz, J. M., Downs, S. H., Leuenberger, P., Ackermann-Liebrich, U. (2006). Prevalence of renal impairment and its association with cardiovascular risk factors in a general population: results of the Swiss SAPALDIA study. *Nephrol Dial Transplant, 21*(4), 935-944.

Pereira, A. A., Weiner, D. E., Scott, T., Chandra, P., Bluestein, R., Griffith, J., & Sarnak, M. J. (2007). Subcortical cognitive impairment in dialysis patients. *Hemodial Int, 11*(3), 309-314.

Pereira, A. A., Weiner, D. E., Scott, T., & Sarnak, M. J. (2005). Cognitive function in dialysis patients. *American Journal of Kidney Diseases, 45*(3), 448-462.

Pinsky, B. W., Takemoto, S. K., Lentine, K. L., Burroughs, T. E., Schnitzler, M. A., & Salvalaggio, P. R. (2009). Transplant Outcomes and Economic Costs Associated with Patient Noncompliance to Immunosuppression. *American Journal of Transplantation, 9*(11), 2597-2606.

Ponton, P., Rupolo, G. P., Marchini, F., Feltrin, A., Perin, N., Mazzoldi, M. A., Rigotti, P. (2001). Quality-of-life change after kidney transplantation. *Transplantation Proceedings, 33*(1-2), 1887-1889.

Qunibi, W. Y., Barri, Y., Devol, E., Alfurayh, O., Sheth, K., & Taher, S. (1991). Factors Predictive of Posttransplant Erythrocytosis. *Kidney International, 40*(6), 1153-1159.

Radic, J., Ljutic, D., Radic, M., Kovacic, V., Curkovic, K. D., & Sain, M. (2011). Cognitive-Psychomotor Functions and Nutritional Status in Maintenance Hemodialysis Patients: Are They Related? *Therapeutic Apheresis and Dialysis, 15*(6), 532-539.

Radic, J., Ljutic, D., Radic, M., Kovacic, V., Dodig-Curkovic, K., & Sain, M. (2011a). Kidney transplantation improves cognitive and psychomotor functions in adult hemodialysis patients. *Am J Nephrol, 34*(5), 399-406.

Radic, J., Ljutic, D., Radic, M., Kovacic, V., Sain, M., & Curkovic, K. D. (2010). The possible impact of dialysis modality on cognitive function in chronic dialysis patients. [Review]. *Netherlands Journal of Medicine, 68*(4), 153-157.

Radic, J., Ljutic, D., Radic, M., Kovacic, V., Sain, M., & Dodig-Curkovic, K. (2011b). Is There Differences in Cognitive and Motor Functioning between Hemodialysis and Peritoneal Dialysis Patients? *Renal Failure, 33*(6), 641-649.

Sehgal, A. R., Grey, S. F., DeOreo, P. B., & Whitehouse, P. J. (1997). Prevalence, recognition, and implications of mental impairment among hemodialysis patients. *American Journal of Kidney Diseases, 30*(1), 41-49.

Singh, N. P., Sahni, V., Wadhwa, A., Garg, S., Bajaj, S. K., Kohli, R., & Agarwal, S. K. (2006). Effect of improvement in anemia on electroneurophysiological markers (P300) of cognitive dysfunction in chronic kidney disease. *Hemodial Int, 10*(3), 267-273.

Stoehr, G. P., Lu, S. Y., Lavery, L., Bilt, J. V., Saxton, J. A., Chang, C. C. H., & Ganguli, M. (2008). Factors Associated with Adherence to Medication Regimens in Older Primary Care Patients: The Steel Valley Seniors Survey. *American Journal of Geriatric Pharmacotherapy, 6*(5), 255-263. Suthanthiran, M., & Strom, T. B. (1994). Medical Progress - Renal-Transplantation. *New England Journal of Medicine, 331*(6), 365-376.

Teschan, P. E., Ginn, H. E., Bourne, J. R., & Ward, J. W. (1976). Neurobehavioral Responses to Middle Molecule Dialysis and Transplantation. *Transactions American Society for Artificial Internal Organs, 22*, 190-194.

Tilki, H. E., Akpolat, T., Tunali, G., Kara, A., & Onar, M. K. (2004). Effects of haemodialysis and continuous ambulatory peritoneal dialysis on P300 cognitive potentials in uraemic patients. *Ups J Med Sci, 109*(1), 43-48.

Tonelli, M., Wiebe, N., Knoll, G., Bello, A., Browne, S., Jadhav, D., Gill, J. (2011). Systematic Review: Kidney Transplantation Compared With Dialysis in Clinically Relevant Outcomes. *American Journal of Transplantation, 11*(10), 2093-2109.

Umans, J. G., & Pliskin, N. H. (1998). Attention and mental processing speed in hemodialysis patients. *American Journal of Kidney Diseases, 32*(5), 749-751.

Wolcott, D. L., Wellisch, D. K., Marsh, J. T., Schaeffer, J., Landsverk, J., & Nissenson, A. R. (1988). Relationship of dialysis modality and other factors to cognitive function in chronic dialysis patients. *Am J Kidney Dis, 12*(4), 275-284.

CHAPTER 7

Treatment Adherence in Patients Undergoing Dialysis

Alden Y. Lai[1] and Konstadina Griva[2,*]

[1]*Graduate School of Medicine, School of Public Health, The University of Tokyo, Tokyo, Japan and* [2]*Faculty of Arts & Social Sciences, Department of Psychology, National University of Singapore, Singapore*

Abstract: Patient non-adherence is a pertinent issue as it induces adverse disease outcomes, poor prognosis, and diminished quality of life. Concerns for non-adherence are further pronounced in End-Stage Kidney Disease (ESKD) patients as treatment is highly complex and demanding with dialysis sessions, multiple medications, and lifestyle restrictions related to dietary and fluid management. Summarising literature on adherence in dialysis patients, this chapter starts by introducing the treatment rationale and regime for ESKD patients undergoing dialysis, followed by a delineation of relevant measures and criteria related to, and rates of non-adherence. An assortment of methods is being used to assess adherence rates in dialysis patients, among which the examining of biochemical markers and patient self-report are the most prevalent. Rates of non-adherence in dialysis patients warrant urgent attention as they can be as high as 18% for missed dialysis sessions, 22.4% for shortened treatment time, 80.4% for medication, 75.3% for fluid restrictions and 81.4% for dietary restrictions. There is a disproportionate emphasis on haemodialysis over peritoneal patients. Paramount to drive efforts to improve treatment adherence in this patient population, demographic, clinical and psychosocial determinants of non-adherence are also highlighted. This chapter concludes with a brief overview on educational and psycho-educational interventions used to improve treatment adherence in patients undergoing dialysis.

Keywords: End-stage kidney disease, kidney failure, dialysis, adherence, compliance, haemodialysis, peritoneal, diet, fluid, medication.

TREATMENT ADHERENCE IN DIALYSIS

The World Health Organization (WHO) defines adherence as "the extent to which a person's behaviour - taking medications, following a recommended diet, and/or executing lifestyle changes, corresponds to the agreed recommendations of a

*Address correspondence to Konstadina Griva: Faculty of Arts & Social Sciences, Department of Psychology, National University of Singapore, Singapore; Tel: +65 65163156; Fax: +65 6773-1843; E-mail: psygk@nus.edu.sg

health care provider" (Sabate, 2003). Adherence ensures patients receive the maximum benefits of prescribed medical treatments, and is of vital importance due to repercussions on patients' safety, quality of life (QoL), disease outcomes such as increased mortality and hospitalisation risks, which in turn impacts upon healthcare costs and the effectiveness of health systems (Sabate, 2003; van Dulmen *et al.*, 2007). Non-adherence is a widespread and persistent problem in the medical world – a systematic review has concluded adherence rates in chronic disease sufferers in developed countries to be 50% (Haynes, 2001), and this figure is thought to be even lower in developing countries (Sabate, 2003).

Recent academic discourse on adherence has further branched into the distinction between intentional/deliberate and unintentional non-adherence. Intentional non-adherence is thought to be an active, deliberate process such as patients making a decision to deviate from treatment guidelines (*e.g.*, missing/altering medication doses or taking medication at different times or discontinuing medications before prescribed course). Unintentional non-adherence, on the other hand, is not resultant of rational decision making but might be randomly induced by factors beyond patients' control, such as the forgetting of medication intake when patients' routines are disrupted, or when they deviate from treatment recommendations due to misunderstanding or poor communication with health care providers (Wroe, 2002). Factors driving intentional and unintentional adherence have been shown to differ; patients' beliefs, attitudes, values or motivations are thought to underlie deliberate non-adherence (Lehane, & McCarthy, 2007; Unni, & Farris, 2011), while unintentional non-adherence can be attributed to the complexity of treatment regime, certain socio-demographic characteristics, or factors related to health literacy or hospitalisation (Bell *et al.*, 2011; Daleboudt, Broadbent, McQueen, & Kaptein, 2011; Gadkari, & McHorney, 2012; Lindquist *et al.*, 2012; Wroe, 2002).

There has therefore been advocacy to categorise adherence behaviours into either intentional or unintentional so as to identify the underlying mechanisms, thus allowing the design of more effective interventions. However, this approach of differentiating between intentional or non-intentional non-adherence in the context of dialysis patients has not received much attention to date. While the importance of distinguishing between both categories of non-adherence might be noteworthy, for ease of discussion, the WHO's definition of adherence as the incongruence between patients' adherence behaviours to that with treatment recommendations provided by the healthcare provider will serve as the basis in this chapter.

ADHERENCE IN THE CONTEXT OF END-STAGE KIDNEY DISEASE

In chronic kidney disease (CKD), the decline of kidney function is irreversible and progresses gradually, with each degree of functional decline corresponding to a specific stage. The final stage in CKD (stage 5) is typically referred to as End-Stage Kidney Disease (ESKD). In ESKD there is a complete or near-complete loss of kidney function with accumulation of toxins, fluid and waste products, and patients need to start on renal replacement therapy (RRT) either in the form of dialysis or renal transplant to sustain life. Given the limited availability of organ donors and unsuitability of some patients for surgery, the majority of ESKD patients are maintained on dialysis either *via* haemodialysis (HD) or peritoneal dialysis (PD). HD involves the replacement of kidney function *via* diffusion processes between patients' blood and a dialyzer (see Fig. **1**), while PD achieves the same objective with a catheter inserted into the peritoneal cavity (see Fig. **2**). PD further consists of two different forms – Continuous Ambulatory Peritoneal Dialysis (CAPD) and Automatic Peritoneal Dialysis (APD) (Figs. **3** and **4** respectively).

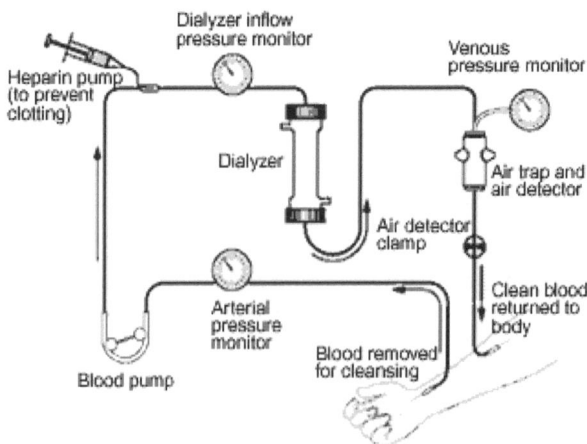

Figure 1: Schematic diagram of HD.

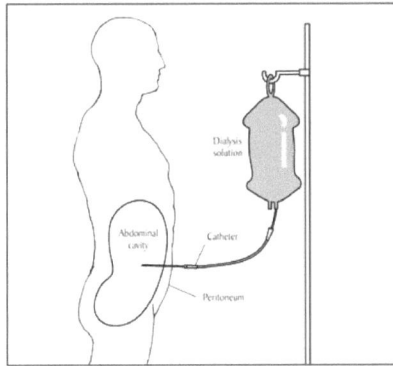

Figure 2: Schematic diagram of PD.

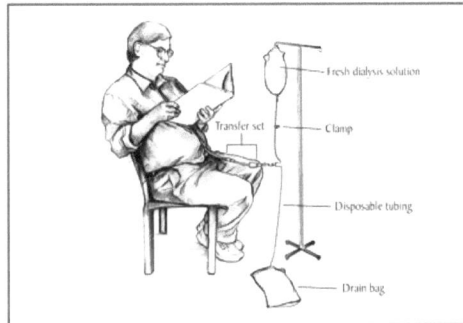

Figure 3: Schematic diagram of CAPD.

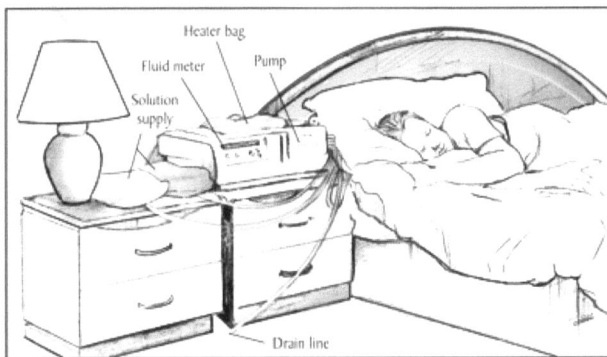

Figure 4: Schematic diagram of APD.

Databases of ESKD epidemiology that are in widespread use include the United States Renal Data System (USRDS) and the UK Renal Registry, which reported 397,796 and 25,796 ESKD patients to undergo either *HD* or PD to sustain their lives in the US and UK respectively in 2009 (Steenkamp, Castledine, Feest, &

Fogarty, 2010; U.S. Renal Data System, 2011). At the global scale, the ESKD population undergoing dialysis was projected to exceed 2 million by 2010 (Lysaght, 2002). These overwhelming figures have shaped research in ESKD patients to almost exclusively emphasise on dialysis patients, explaining the focus of ESRD patients undergoing dialysis in this chapter.

The issue of adherence in dialysis patients is a pertinent one, as dialysis notwithstanding, treatment regimes for ESKD involves a complex and demanding behavioural regimen related to nutritional management (*i.e.,* fluid and diet restrictions), medication and exercise (Sharp, Wild, & Gumley, 2004).

ESKD patients on HD usually undergo tri-weekly sessions at a hospital unit or dialysis centre each lasting four hours approximately, and depending on their treatment mode PD patients perform renal exchanges either four to five times daily (for CAPD), or throughout the night (for APD) (National Kidney Foundation, 2012). Fluid and diet restrictions also form an integral part of the ESKD treatment regime. While specific guidelines differ according to the individual, patients are generally advised to reduce ingestion of foods high in sodium, potassium and phosphorus, and maintain optimal calcium levels as upsetting the mineral/electrolyte balance induces bone demineralisation and metabolic complications, sometimes even life-threatening symptoms (*e.g.,* breathlessness) (National Kidney Foundation, 2010). Fluid restrictions are imposed on dialysis patients due to an inability to produce urine and remove fluid, and an excessive fluid intake can result in pulmonary edema and poses higher cardiovascular risks (Tracy, Green, & McCleary, 1987). In terms of medication, phosphate binders facilitate the intestinal excretion of phosphorus in lieu of the impairment of kidney function to do so, and are the most commonly prescribed form of medication for dialysis patients (Bame, Petersen, & Wray, 1993). Chronic high phosphorus levels affect cardiovascular, blood circulatory and bone health (National Kidney Foundation, 2010; Weed-Collins, & Hogan, 1989), therefore necessitating the routine intake of phosphate binders for ESKD patients.

Dialysis is the lifeline of ESKD patients as it replaces the kidneys' function to extract metabolic wastes. However, other lifestyle adjustments related to nutrition and medication are also vital determinants of ESKD outcomes, henceforth explaining the need to examine the whole spectrum of dialysis patients' adherence behaviours. Non-adherence is a major problem as this regimen has many characteristics that have been shown to decrease adherence – treatment is complex, long lasting and impinges upon multiple domains on patients' lives. For example, research has highlighted dialysis patients to be required to take 10 different prescriptions at various occasions throughout the day (Manley *et al.*, 2004). Furthermore, most patients are typically diagnosed in late adulthood when health behaviours are firmly established, hence additional change is far more challenging and difficult to maintain. The regimen is further complicated by the need to integrate diet and medication regimes for co-existing conditions or ESKD complications such as heart disease, hypertension or diabetes. In light of this, perhaps it should not come as a surprise that a substantial number of patients fail to manage treatment, constituting high non-adherence rates.

Recent reviews have revealed rates of up to 86% of non-adherence to dialysis sessions (Matteson, & Russel, 2010) and 80% for oral medication in HD patients (Schmid, Hartmann, & Schiffl, 2009). A large study also delineated 81.4% and 74.6% of HD patients to harbour difficulties adhering to diet and fluid restrictions respectively (Kugler, Vlaminck, Haverich, & Maes, 2005). The lifestyle aspects of treatment are particularly challenging as patients are required to drastically limit fluid intake and make dietary adjustments that are somewhat unconventional and incompatible with main principles of healthy eating such as foregoing consumption of certain fruits and vegetables or limiting intake of dairy products.

The documented high non-adherence rates are a cause of concern as non-adherence has been shown to be associated with adverse clinical outcomes and poor prognosis which in turn lead to increased costs and expenditure for patient care (Bender, & Rand, 2004; Sokol, McGuigan, Verbrugge, & Epstein, 2005; Sunanda, & Fadia, 2008). There is ample evidence that mortality and mortality are higher in patients who do not follow treatment – skipping dialysis treatments once or more per month has been shown to increase the likelihood of death by 25%, and by 13% for hospitalisation (Leggat, Orzol, & Hulbert-Shearon, 1998; Saran, Bragg-Gresham, & Rayner, 2003). Poor adherence to fluid restrictions was also associated with 35% more risk of death (Leggat, *et al.*, 1998), whereas deficient dietary non-adherence has been linked with 50-59% of increased mortality risks (Unruh, Evans, Fink, Powe, & Meyer, 2005).

Non-adherence may also compromise dialysis patient QoL. ESKD is a chronic disease that impacts upon patients and/or their caregivers due to the demanding nature of self-management regimen and the continuity that is required of it (Killingworth, 1993). Inadequate adherence to nutritional guidelines has been demonstrated to interfere with ESRD patients' QoL, and poor physical and psychological well-being are also correlated with higher risks of death and hospitalisation (Valderrabano, Jofre, & Lopez-Gomez, 2001). The function of QoL as a predictor of mortality, risks of hospitalisation and depression is also well documented in studies with large samples of dialysis patients (DeOreo, 1997; Lopes *et al.*, 2003; Mapes *et al.*, 2003). Psychosocial factors, such as a perceived lack of social support from family and friends, feelings of isolation and as a burden are further associated with compromised adherence rates (Untas *et al.*, 2011). As adverse effects or symptoms of non-adherence can impinge upon domains spanning across physical, psychological and social aspects in dialysis patients, the study of adherence in chronic diseases like ESKD remains a justified agenda.

The recognition of magnitude of problem and dire consequences in terms of clinical management and health care has led to burgeoning research interest in the development and evaluation of intervention programs to support behavioural change in the context of dialysis and increase adherence rates. Literature on studies aiming to increase adherence in dialysis patients have been uprising since the last few decades. Following an outline of measurement methods, definitions, rates and determinants of non-adherence in dialysis patients *via* selected studies, this chapter will present a brief overview of the interventions and their underlying methodologies that have been implemented to improve ESKD patients' levels of adherence.

MEASURES OF NON-ADHERENCE IN DIALYSIS

As the treatment regime for dialysis patients' spans across domains of both medical and lifestyle components, studies investigating dialysis patients' adherence are also hugely diverse in terms of measurement methods and definitions of adherence. Adherence behaviours in dialysis patients are usually categorised into domains related to attendance at dialysis sessions, medication intake, and complying with fluid and diet restrictions.

Biochemical data obtained from clinical measurements are widely used to measure adherence in dialysis patients. Typical biochemical markers of renal adherence include pre-dialysis serum phosphate (SP), which is used mostly as an indicator of medication adherence; pre-dialysis serum potassium (SK), mostly to assess diet adherence, and inter-dialytic weight gain (IDWG) as a measurement of fluid restriction. SP and SK serve as indicators of medication and diet adherence, as the loss of kidney function parallels diminished abilities to excrete phosphorus and potassium, henceforth dialysis patients are required to take phosphate binders during mealtimes to facilitate the excretion of phosphorus from their body and are advised to limit foods with high-potassium content. It is crucial to consider however, while SP is a typically used as a marker of adherence to medication, it can also be influenced by other factors such as residual kidney function, dietary adherence and dialysis attendance (Schmid, *et al.*, 2009). SP and SK are therefore not specific to a particular domain in ESKD treatment adherence; elevated levels may reflect dietary non-adherence and/or lapses in medication intake.

IDWG, generally defined as the gain in body weight post-dialysis, gives an indication of the degree of adherence to fluid restrictions given the kidneys' incapability to regulate fluid levels. High weight gains (calculated either as simple pre to post weight gain formulae or more complex/tailored calculations to account for BMI or body weight) indicate excessive fluid intake across dialysis sessions.

Assessing these biochemical markers of adherence *via* reviews of medical records is thus highly prevalent in adherence research in the context of dialysis patients, although definitions of non-adherence vary. Cut-off values for these markers differ however – non-adherence to medication was defined as an SP value of > 4.59 mg/dL (Lin, & Liang, 1997), 5.5 mg/dL (Khalil, Frazier, Lennie, & Sawaya, 2011; Tomasello, Dhupar, & Sherman, 2004), 6.0 mg/dL (Lin, & Liang, 1997), or 7.5 mg/dL (Hecking *et al.*, 2004; Kutner, Zhang, McClellan, & Cole, 2002; Leggat, *et al.*, 1998; Saran, *et al.*, 2003). An SK value of above 5.5 (Khalil, *et al.*, 2011), 6.0

(Hecking, *et al.*, 2004; Saran, *et al.*, 2003) or 6.5 mg/dL (Bame, *et al.*, 1993) has been used as the threshold value in defining diet non-adherence. For non-adherence to fluid restrictions, definitions of IDWG > 1.0kg/day (Bame, *et al.*, 1993), >3.5% (Lindberg, Prutz, Lindberg, & Wikstrom, 2009) or >5.7% of dry weight (Hecking, *et al.*, 2004; Leggat, *et al.*, 1998; Lindberg, *et al.*, 2009; Saran, *et al.*, 2003) have been observed. The unit of measurement was also not standardised, as seen from Lee and Molassiotis (2002)'s usage of SP> 2.0mmol/l and SK> 5.5mmol/l as indicators of medication and diet non-adherence respectively. Finally, only a few studies reflected the usage of blood urea nitrogen (BUN) as an indicator of diet adherence (Bame, *et al.*, 1993; Khalil, *et al.*, 2011). Such inconsistencies in definitions were posed to be a major obstacle in assessment of and research on adherence in dialysis patients (Denhaerynck *et al.*, 2007).

Apart from the assessment/recording of biochemical markers, a range of other measures have been employed across studies, including patient self-report, Medication Events Monitoring System (MEMS®), nurse/nephrologist assessments to inventory checks. Patient self-report was the mostly utilised mode of assessment, as information on adherence behaviours is difficult to obtain without soliciting information from patients. Non-adherence to dialysis sessions was classified into either missed or shortened treatments, therefore patient self-report on adherence to dialysis treatments typically include questions directly assessing frequencies of skipped dialysis treatments and the duration of the shortening of sessions. There is seemingly a consensus on study definitions regarding non-adherence to dialysis sessions – missed sessions were defined as absence of one or more session per month, and shortened treatments were defined as shortening dialysis by 10 minutes or more in at least one or more session per month (Hecking, *et al.*, 2004; Leggat, *et al.*, 1998; Saran, *et al.*, 2003). On the other hand, questions pertaining to adherence to medication, and fluid and diet restrictions probe the missed amount of medication dosage and patients' perception of the degree of their fluid and/or diet restrictions (Cleary, Matzke, Alexander, & Joy, 1995; Lee, & Molassiotis, 2002; Rahman, & Griffin, 2004; Tomasello, *et al.*, 2004). Kimmel *et al.*, (1995) and Lindberg *et al.*, (1997) have further examined the discrepancies between patient self-report against that of clinician-prescribed medication list or recommended dialysis duration for reinforced data on dialysis patients' adherence levels. The use of technological devices to measure non-adherence, such as MEMS®, allows the capture of information on dates and times of the opening of medication bottles, and measurements of under dosing, overdosing, or days when medication were not taken (Curtin, Svarstad, Andress, Keller, & Sacksteder, 1997; Curtin, Svarstad, & Keller, 1999). Curtin *et al.,* (1997) and Curtin *et al.,* (1999) utilised MEMS® in their studies and defined medication non-adherence as missing 20% or more of prescribed dosage. Fine (1997) used inventory checks to measure non-adherence, and defined non-adherence to PD sessions as using less than 90% of prescribed dialysate solution.

Two self-report instruments measuring non-adherence in dialysis patients – the Dialysis Diet and Fluid Non-adherence Questionnaire (DDFQ) (Vlaminck, Maes, Jacobs, Reyntjens, & Evers, 2001) and Morisky Medication Adherence Scale (MMAS) (Morisky, Green, & Levine, 1986) were commonly used to assess non-adherence to fluid and diet restrictions, or medication in a number of studies (Kara, Caglar, & Kilic, 2007; Kugler, Maeding, & Russel, 2011; Kugler, *et al.*, 2005; Neri *et al.*, 2011; Rahman & Griffin, 2004; Vlaminck, *et al.*, 2001). The four-item DDFQ consists of two subscales to measure diet and fluid non-adherence each, assessing the frequency of non-adherence behaviour in the previous 14 days and the perceived severity of deviation from one's treatment recommendations. Perceived degree for non-adherence is scored on a 5-point Likert scale, with '0' for 'no deviation' and '5' for 'very severe deviation'. The four-item MMAS, while not developed specifically to dialysis patients, measures non-adherence to medication with four close-ended questions with binary responses and has been widely used in other patient populations.

The Simplified Medication Adherence Questionnaire (SMAQ) is also a tool which evaluates patient's adherence. It is a short and simple tool based on questions posed directly to the patient regarding his/her medication-taking habits (Theofilou, 2012a), which was originally validated for the measurement of adherence in patients on anti-retroviral treatment (Knobel, Alonso, Casado, Collazos, Gonzalez *et al.*, 2002). In the field of nephrology, this tool has been used for evaluating compliance with phosphate-binding treatment in haemodialysis patients, although it has not been validated for this group of patients. This questionnaire consists of six questions that evaluate different aspects of patient compliance with treatment: forgetfulness, routine, adverse effects, and a quantification of omissions (Theofilou, 2012a). A patient is classified as non-compliant if he/she responds to any of the questions with a non-adherence answer, and in terms of quantification, if the patient has lost more than two doses during the last week or has not taken medication during more than two complete days during the last three months.

With manifold components in the ESKD treatment regime, it is essential to have standardised measurements of dialysis patients' adherence. Kaveh *et al.*, (2001) underlined the lack of a standardised paradigm to examine adherence in ESKD patients, proffering a 'gold standard' of multidimensional measures of adherence related to dialysis sessions, medication, diet, bio-clinical markers, simultaneously highlighting the need to also consider psychosocial variables. The Kidney Disease Outcomes Quality Initiative (KDOQI) Clinical Practice Guidelines – a set of extensively used recommendations developed by the National Kidney Foundation – further delineated measures of non-adherence as missed or shortened dialysis sessions, IDWG, SK, serum albumin and treatment adequacy (Kt/V) (Colette, Wazny, & Sood, 2011). These adherence indices can together serve as benchmarks for the evaluation of dialysis patients' adherence levels. However, as seen from above, these recommendations have yet to be fully integrated, as observed from the lack of studies including variables such of serum albumin or Kt/V in the studies. The challenge to develop a set of comprehensive framework to assess adherence levels in research with dialysis patients therefore remains.

RATES OF NON-ADHERENCE IN DIALYSIS

Table **1** provides an overview of selected studies examining rates of non-adherence in dialysis patients.

Table 1: Overview of selected studies of treatment adherence in dialysis patient.

Study	Year	Type of Dialysis (N)	Location of Study	Rate of Non-adherence (%)					Mode of assessment	Definition of Non-adherence
				Dialysis treatment		Medication	Fluid	Diet		
				Missed	Shortened					
Bame et al.,	1993	HD (1230)	US	-	-	50.2	49.5	2-9	Review of medical records	SK > 6.5 mEq/dL; SP > 6.0mg/dL; BUN > 100mg/dL; IDWG > 1.0kg/day
Cleary et al.,	1995	HD (51) CAPD (21)	US	-	-	52 (HD) 50 (PD)	-	-	Patient self-report	Missed medication dose
Kimmel et al.,	1995	HD (149)	US	0-17.9	0-22.4	-	-	-	Patient self-report	Discrepancy between actual time on HD and prescribed duration
Lin et al.,	1997	HD (86)	Taiwan	-	-	61	-	-	Patient self-report Nurse assessment	SP > 4.59 mg/dL
Curtin et al.,	1997	HD (135)	US	-	-	42-80	-	-	MEMS	Missing 20% ≥ prescribed dose
Fine	1997	PD (93)	Canada	12-15	-	-	-	-	Inventory checks	Using < 90% of prescribed dialysate
Leggat et al.,	1998	HD (6251)	US	8.5	20	22	10	-	Secondary analysis of data from medical records	Missing ≥ 1 session/month Shortening by 10min ≥ in 1 or more session/month IDWG ≥ 5.7% of dry weight SP > 7.5mg/dL
Bernardini et al.,	1998	PD (49)	US	35	-	-	-	-	Inventory check	No. of exchanges performed/no. prescribed
Curtin et al.,	1999	HD (135)	US	-	-	73	-	-	MEMS	Over/underdose; missing ≥ 20% of prescribed dosage
Bleyer et al.,	1999	HD (693)	Multinational	0-2.3	-	-	-	-	Nurse/Nephrologist Assessment	Missed dialysis sessions
Blake et al.,	2000	PD (656)	US Canada	13	-	-	-	-	Patient self-report	Missed ≥ 1 dialysis/week, or ≥ 2 dialysis/month

Table 1: contd....

Study	Year	Sample	Country						Method	Definition
Vlaminck et al.,	2001	HD (564)	Belgium	-	-	-	72	81.4	Patient self-report	Dialysis Diet and Fluid Non-adherence Questionnaire
Pang et al.,	2001	HD (92)	Hong Kong	-	-	-	32.6	-	Review of medical records	IDWG > 0.9kg/day
Kutner et al.,	2002	HD (119) PD (59)	US	18 (HD) 30 (PD)	31 (HD)	19 (HD) 10 (PD)	-	-	Review of medical records	SP > 7.5mg/dL
Lee et al.,	2002	HD (62)	Hong Kong	-	-	56.5	69.7	38.7	Patient self-report Review of medical Records	Perceived degree of fluid/diet adherence during past week (0-7; >4 = adherent) SK > 5.5mmol/l SP > 2.0 mmol/l IDWG > 0.7kg/day (for total weight < 50kg) and 1.0kg/day (for total weight > 50kg)
Saran et al.,	2003	HD (7676)	Multinational	3.8	13	13.7	19.6	10.8	Review of medical records	SK > 6.0 mEq/dL SP > 7.5mg/dL IDWG > 5.7% of dry weight Missing ≥ 1 dialysis session/month Shortening by ≥ 10 min in 1 or more session/month
Tomasello et al.,	2004	HD (129) PD (59)	US	-	-	37.8	-	-	Patient self-report Review of medical Records	Missing 20% or more of prescribed dose SP > 5.5mg/dL
Rahman et al.,	2004	HD (270)	US	-	-	23	-	-	Patient self-report	Morisky Medication Adherence Scale
Hecking et al.,	2004	HD (3039)	Multinational	0.6	9	-	9.8	18	Review of medical records	SK > 6.0 mEq/dL SP > 7.5mg/dL IDWG > 5.7% of body weight Missing ≥ 1 dialysis session/month Shortening by ≥ 10 min in 1 or more session/month

Table 1: contd….

Author	Year	Sample	Country						Method	Instrument
Kugler et al.,	2005	HD (916)	Germany Belgium	-	-	-	74.6	81.4	Patient self-report	Dialysis Diet and Fluid Non-adherence Questionnaire
Holley et al.,	2006	HD (39) PD(15)	US	-	-	18 - 21	-	-	Patient self-report	Reasons for not taking medication
Lindberg et al.,	2007	HD (144) PD (60)	Sweden	-	-	80.4	-	-	Patient self-report Medication prescription	Discrepancy between self-reported rates and medication prescriptions
Kara et al.,	2007	HD (160)	Turkey	-	-	-	68.1	58.1	Patient self-report	Dialysis Diet and Fluid Non-adherence Questionnaire
Hirth et al.,	2008	HD (5438)	Multinational	-	-	3 - 29	-	-	Patient self-report	Cost-related non-adherence
Lam et al.,	2009	CAPD (173)	Hong Kong	7		17	36	72	Structured interviews	Dialysis Diet and Fluid Non-adherence Questionnaire
Lindberg et al.,	2009	HD (4498)	Sweden	-	-	-	4.8 - 31.5	-	Secondary analysis of data from medical records	IDWG > 3.5% of body weight IDWG > 5.7% of body weight
Kugler et al.,	2011	HD (495)	US Germany	-	-	-	75.3	80.4	Patient self-report	Dialysis Diet and Fluid Non-adherence Questionnaire
Khalil et al.,	2011	HD (100)	US	-	-	9 - 50	44 - 56		Patient self-report Review of medical reports	Dialysis Diet and Fluid Non-adherence Questionnaire SK > 5.5mg/dL SP > 5.5mg/dL BUN > 100mg/dL
Neri et al.,	2011	HD (1238)	Italy	-	-	52	-	-	Patient self-report	Morisky Medication Adherence Scale

As evident from these selected studies, there is a high degree of variance in non-adherence levels, ranging from 0-18% for missed dialysis sessions, 0-22.4% for shortened treatment time, 3-80.4% for medication, 9.8-75.3% for fluid intake, and 2-81.4% for diet restrictions. Despite the huge variance, the upper limits of these figures, especially those of non-adherence to fluid and diet restrictions, and medication in this patient population certainly warrant urgent attention. Appropriate medication intake, and following fluid and diet restrictions can thus be inferred to pose more difficulties in adherence over dialysis treatments itself in dialysis patients.

In terms of coverage of the various adherence behaviours, only Saran *et al.,* (2003) and Lam, Twinn and Chan (2010)'s studies simultaneously delved into all four domains of adherence behaviours, while Bame *et al.,* (1993), Lee and Molassiotis (2002) and Leggat *et al.,* (1998) examined a combination of three out of the four. The number of participants in these studies also spanned between 49 and 7,676, constituting a probable explanation for the large variance in results.

In contrast to HD, very few studies have explored adherence in PD patients (Bernardini, & Piraino, 1998; Blake *et al.,* 2000; Fine, 1997; Lam, *et al.,* 2010), indicating a need for more research in this dialysis population. Non-adherence to peritoneal exchanges is the aspect that was most researched in this population, whereas little attention has been given on the lifestyle aspects of the regimen, namely diet or medication. Rates of non-adherence to PD exchanges have been shown to range between 7-35%. In the largest study to date (N=656) by Blake *et al.,* (2000), a total 13% of PD patients were found to be non-adherent to dialysis exchanges based on a definition of missing one or more dialysis session per week, or two or more per month.

None of the identified studies measured adherence to physical activity. Exercise is widely recommended for patients on dialysis as it improves clinical and psychological outcomes. The beneficial effects of exercise on dialysis patients, include enhanced dialysis outcomes, better QoL, nutritional status, and physiological improvements such as muscular strength, peak oxygen consumption and heart rate variability (Cheema, Smith, & Singh, 2005; Segura-Orti, & Johansen, 2010; Smart, & Steele, 2011). Intradialytic exercise programmes, when conducted appropriately, have been advocated in dialysis patients due to the abundance of benefits it induces with minimal safety concerns (Brenner, 2009). The lack of research on adherence to exercise regimes or physical activity recommendations in dialysis patients should therefore be noted to propel further studies in this particular area.

DETERMINANTS OF NON-ADHERENCE IN DIALYSIS

In delineating rates of non-adherence, it is crucial to simultaneously note the determinants of non-adherence in dialysis patients. A recent systematic review of 34 studies conducted by Karamanidou *et al.,* on non-adherence to phosphate-binding medication in ESKD patients categorised determinants into either demographic, clinical or psychosocial factors (Karamanidou, Clatworthy, Weinman, & Horne, 2008). Demographic predictors that were significant in predicting medication non-adherence included age, education, marital status/living arrangement, ethnic group and income; those clinically related were identified to be duration on dialysis, diabetic status, transplant history and complexity of regimen. Psychosocial variables – *i.e.,* health beliefs, personality characteristics, health locus of control, social support, family dynamics, knowledge, and anxiety/depression – were however concluded to have stronger associations with ESKD patients' medication non-adherence as compared with demographic and clinical variables in this review. In a separate review conducted earlier, Loghman-Adham (2003) also similarly inferred complexity of regimen, ethnic group, age, education, family dynamics, and psychosocial factors as predictors of medication non-adherence in dialysis patients. Among the demographic factors, being younger in age has been identified as a consistent predictor of non-adherence (Bame, *et al.*, 1993; Leggat, 2005; Leggat, *et al.*, 1998; Russell, Knowles, & Peace, 2007).

An abundance of literature exists on the association between depression/depressive symptoms and non-adherence in dialysis patients. DeOreo (1997) conducted a study with 1,000 HD patients and observed patients with lower perceived mental health levels to exhibit a likelihood for hospitalisation, and to skip two or more dialysis sessions per month. A systematic review that analysed 44 articles concluded an association between depressive symptoms and dietary non-adherence (Khalil, & Frazier, 2010). This behavioural association is one of the two pathways (the other being biological) that have been underlined to explain the mechanisms behind depressive symptoms and poor disease outcomes in ESKD patients (Khalil, & Frazier, 2010). In addition to depressive symptoms, other psychosocial factors such as health beliefs related to potential side effects, health locus of control, subjective norms, self-efficacy, and perceived benefits of and barriers to medication have also been lined to non- adherence. These cognitions are also highly modifiable constructs that should be targeted in interventions aiming to improve adherence (Theofilou 2012; Horne, Weinman, Barber, Elliott, & Morgan, 2005; Karamanidou, Clatworthy, *et al.*, 2008; Kammerer, Garry, Hartigan, Carter, & Erlich, 2007; Karamanidou, Clatworthy, *et al.*, 2008a).

Apart from demographic, clinical and psychosocial factors, financial cost can also act as barrier to medication intake. International data on 7,776 HD patients across 12 industrialised countries showed cost-related non-adherence rates to be between 3-29. In another study, 67% of patients who chose not to re-fill their medication prescription quoted financial issues as their main reason (Holley, & DeVore, 2006).

INTERVENTIONS TO IMPROVE ADHERENCE

In the context of poor adherence rates in dialysis patients, various interventions have been conducted in a bid to improve adherence levels.

Intervention work on this patient group is growing, although evidence on their effectiveness is still considerably limited due to concerns related to statistical power, reliability of measurements, limited or short follow-up assessments, and lack of theoretical frameworks. It is also not clear if the value of programs translate or manifest into objective clinical improvements (van Dulmen, *et al.*, 2007; Welch, & Thomas-Hawkins, 2005).

Four systematic reviews related to interventions in dialysis patients have been identified; Welch and Thomas-Hawkins (2005) performed a review of nine psycho-education intervention studies seeking to improve fluid adherence,

Matteson and Russell (2010) reviewed eight randomised controlled trials (RCTs) relevant to improving general patient adherence, Sharp *et al.,* (2005) evaluated 16 psychological studies on improvement for fluid adherence, while Idier, Untas, Koleck, Chauveau and Rascle (2011) assessed 35 articles related to therapeutic patient education. Apparent from the reviews are how interventions in dialysis patients tend to employ either purely a patient educational, or psycho-educational approach – the latter having psychosocial component(s) in addition to the educational segment. Secondly, there has been an emphasis on improving specifically fluid or medication adherence. The systematic reviews have generally concluded interventions to have a substantial extent of success in improving adherence levels in HD patients, although a general consensus on the best intervention strategy has yet to emerge. In addition, these identified reviews have exclusively focussed on intervention studies in the context of HD patients, suggesting an immense lack of research on interventions and/or their effects on PD patients' adherence and outcomes.

Patient educational approaches are fundamentally propelled by the belief that a lack of knowledge leads to poor adherence, as patients either have insufficient understanding on the pertinence of being adherent to their renal treatment regime, or do not possess the know-how to do so. In this vein, patient educational interventions typically focus on increasing patients' awareness of (a) the rationale of certain adherence behaviours, (b) the underlying physiological mechanisms, and (c) adverse disease outcomes associated with non-adherence. To provide an example, contents in the context of phosphate binders included: what are phosphate binders, why the need to take them, how it helps in excreting phosphate compounds out of the body, and how chronic phosphatemia can lead to bone mineral disorders (van Camp, Huybrechts, van Rompaey, & Elseviers, 2011). Patient educational approaches have been demonstrated to increase HD/renal knowledge and have been associated with increased adherence in dialysis patients (Baraz, Parvardeh, Mohammaadi, & Broumand, 2010). However, the effectiveness of patient educational strategies is still questionable as some studies have also highlighted the absence of relationship between reinforcing one's knowledge and their adherence levels (Wells, 2011).

By boosting patient educational interventions with a psychosocial component, psycho-educational strategies have gained attention as approaches to undertake. Psycho-educational interventions in dialysis patients comprise a primary goal to improve adherence and QoL for better self-management of disease, and a secondary aim for enhanced collaboration with caregivers (Idier, *et al.*, 2011). As the term suggests, psycho-educational interventions integrate psychological interventions and educational programmes. These studies can be based on psychological theories or frameworks – Tsay (2003) conducted an intervention with 62 HD patients using Bandura's self-efficacy theory, and Karamanidou, Weinman and Horne (2008a) performed a study with 39 HD patients following Leventhal's self-regulation model. Both studies demonstrated significant results in improved adherence to fluid and medication post-intervention respectively. Sharp, Wild and Gumley (2005a) also employed a cognitive-behavioural approach in 56 HD patients, showing fluid adherence to improve over time. Theory-driven interventions therefore show a degree of promise to guide the formulation of studies to improve adherence in dialysis patients. Nevertheless, interventions based on clearly delineated theories are still scarce, thus rigorous theoretical frameworks and methodologies in its conception are called for (van Dulmen, *et al.*, 2007; Welch, & Thomas-Hawkins, 2005).

Lastly, it is also worth mentioning that renal nurses most often fulfilled the role as interventionists, and this has prompted several intervention studies to advocate them as ideal facilitators of adherence interventions in dialysis patients (Barnett, Li Yoong, Pinikahana, & Si-Yen, 2008; Tsay, 2003; van Camp, *et al.*, 2011). Nurses are in an excellent position to fulfill such roles as they have opportunities to build long-term relationships with patients, simultaneously providing education and encouragement in a continuous manner (Barnett, *et al.*, 2008). They serve as an exemplar to psycho-educational approaches, as renal nurses also have the capacity to counsel patients (*i.e.,* fulfilling the psychological component), yet provide a constant source of information related to ESKD and its treatment (*i.e.,* patient education) for reinforced adherence (van Camp, *et al.*, 2011). Thus, as much as the contents of interventions should be duly considered, efforts to improve adherence should also take into account the role and attributes of interventionists.

CONCLUSIONS

The issue of patient adherence is highly consequential due to its proximal adverse impact on disease outcomes and QoL, and distally healthcare expenditure and effectiveness of health systems. Dialysis patients are a unique patient population in the context of treatment adherence research due to a highly complex treatment regime that concerns multiple facets of their lives; an integration of multiple domains related to dialysis treatment, medication, fluid and diet intake is necessary for optimal disease management. Given this complexity, an assortment of measurement methods, including biochemical markers, patient self-report, technological devices, assessments by healthcare professionals and inventory checks, together with diverse definitions, have been used to examine non-adherence in dialysis patients. Coupled with differing sample sizes, the rates of non-adherence in dialysis patients have a certain degree of variation. Nevertheless, if the upper limits of non-adherence rates were to be considered, especially those pertaining to medication, and fluid and diet restrictions, research findings have converged to accentuate how non-adherence in dialysis patients is a pressing issue. Identifying determinants of non-adherence in this patient population is paramount to drive efforts to support patients and improve adherence to treatment.

This chapter has therefore outlined the broad categories of demographic, clinical and psychosocial factors affecting treatment adherence, and further offered a brief overview on the two main types of interventions (*i.e.,* educational or psycho-educational) used to improve patient adherence.

There are however still issues that have been overlooked and warranted further work. These include a disproportionate emphasis on HD over PD patients, and the lack of studies examining adherence to recommendations related to physical activity.

In summary, this chapter focused on the topic of treatment adherence in patients undergoing dialysis, outlining recent conceptualisation approached, relevant measures and criteria, and summarising literature on adherence rates and determinants, further offering a brief overview of related interventions.

These issues should serve as platform to increase an understanding in this area, and spur additional research that will reinforce adherence rates in this patient population.

ACKNOWLEDGEMENTS

None Declared.

CONFLICT OF INTEREST

None Declared.

REFERENCES

Bame, S. I., Petersen, N., & Wray, N. P. (1993). Variation in hemodialysis patient compliance according to demographic characteristics. Soc Sci Med, 37(8), 1035-1043.

Baraz, S., Parvardeh, S., Mohammaadi, E., & Broumand, B. (2010). Dietary and fluid compliance: an educational intervention for patients having haemodialysis. Journal of Advanced Nursing, 66(1), 60-68.

Barnett, T., Li Yoong, T., Pinikahana, J., & Si-Yen, T. (2008). Fluid compliance among patients having haemodialysis: can an educational programme make a difference? [Evaluation Studies]. Journal of Advanced Nursing, 61(3), 300-306. doi: 10.1111/j.1365-2648.2007.04528.x

Bell, C. M., Brener, S. S., Gunraj, N., Huo, C., Bierman, A. S., Scales, D. C., Urbach, D. R. (2011). Association of ICU or hospital admission with unintentional discontinuation of medications for chronic diseases. The Journal of the American Medical Association, 306(8), 840-847.

Bender, B., & Rand, C. (2004). Medication non-adherence and asthma treatment cost. Current Opinion in Allergy & Clinical Immunology, 4(3), 191-195.

Bernardini, J., & Piraino, B. (1998). Compliance in CAPD and CCPD patients as measured by supply inventories during home visits. American Journal of Kidney Disease, 31(1), 101-107.

Blake, P. G., Korbet, S. M., Blake, R., Bargman, J. M., Burkart, J. M., Delano, B. G., Heidenheim, P. (2000). A multicenter study of noncompliance with continuous ambulatory peritoneal dialysis exchanges in US and Canadian patients. American Journal of Kidney Disease, 35(3), 506-514.

Brenner, I. (2009). Exercise performance by hemodialysis patients: a review of the literature. Phys Sportsmed, 37(4), 84-96.

Cheema, B. S., Smith, B. C., & Singh, M. A. (2005). A rationale for intradialytic exercise training as standard clinical practice in ESRD. Am J Kidney Dis, 45(5), 912-916.

Cleary, D. J., Matzke, G. R., Alexander, A. C., & Joy, M. S. (1995). Medication knowledge and compliance among patients receiving long-term dialysis. American Journal of Health-system pharmacy, 52(17), 1895-1900.

Colette, R. B., Wazny, L. D., & Sood, A. R. (2011). Medication adherence in patients with chronic kidney disease. The CAANT Journal, 21(2), 47-51.

Curtin, R. B., Svarstad, B. L., Andress, D., Keller, T., & Sacksteder, P. (1997). Differences in older *versus* younger, hemodialysis patients' noncompliance with oral medications. Geriatr Nephrol Urol, 7(1), 35-44.

Curtin, R. B., Svarstad, B. L., & Keller, T. (1999). Hemodialysis patients' noncompliance with oral medications. ANNA journal / American Nephrology Nurses' Association, 26(3), 307-316.

Daleboudt, G. M. N., Broadbent, E., McQueen, F., & Kaptein, A. A. (2011). Intentional and unintentional treatment nonadherence in patients with systematic lupus erythematosus. Arthritis care & research, 63(3), 342-350.

Denhaerynck, K., Manhaeve, D., Dobbels, F., Garzoni, D., Nolte, C., & De Geest, S. (2007). Prevalence and consequences of nonadherence to hemodialysis regimens. [Review]. American journal of critical care: an official publication, American Association of Critical-Care Nurses, 16(3), 222-235; quiz 236.

DeOreo, P. B. (1997). Hemodialysis patient-assessed functional health status predicts continued survival, hospitalization, and dialysis-attendance compliance. American Journal of Kidney Disease, 30(2), 204-212.

Fine, A. (1997). Compliance with CAPD prescription is good. Perit Dial Dial, 17(4), 343-346.

Gadkari, A. S., & McHorney, C. A. (2012). Unintentional non-adherence to chronic prescription medications: how unintentional is it really? BMC health services research, 12(98).

Haynes, R. B. (2001). Interventions for helping patients to follow prescriptions for medications. Cochrane database of systematic reviews(1).

Hecking, E., Bragg-Gresham, J. L., Rayner, H. C., Pisoni, R. L., Andreucci, V. E., Combe, C., Port, F. K. (2004). Haemodialysis prescription, adherence and nutritional indicators in five European countries: results from the Dialysis Outcomes and Practice Patterns Study (DOPPS). Nephro Dial Transplant, 19(1), 100-107.

Hirth, R. A., Greer, S. L., Albert, J. M., Young, E. W., & Piette, J.D. (2008). Out-of-pocket spending and medication adherence among dialysis patients in twelve countries. Health affairs, 27(1), 89-102.

Holley, J. L., & DeVore, C. C. (2006). Why all prescribed medications are not taken: results from a survey of chronic dialysis patients. Adv Perit Dial, 22, 162-166.

Horne, R., Weinman, J., Barber, N., Elliott, R. A., & Morgan, M. (2005). Concordance, adherence and compliance in medicine taking: a conceptual map and research priorities. London: National Co-ordinating Centre for NHS Service Delivery and Organisation NCCSDO.

Idier, L., Untas, A., Koleck, M., Chauveau, P., & Rascle, N. (2011). Assessment and effects of Therapeutic Patient Education for patients in hemodialysis: A systematic review. International Journal of Nursing Studies, 48(12), 1570-1586.

Kammerer, N., Garry, G., Hartigan, M., Carter, B., & Erlich, L. (2007). Adherence in patients on dialysis: strategies for success. Nephrology Nursing Journal, 34(5), 479-486.

Kara, B., Caglar, K., & Kilic, S. (2007). Nonadherence with diet and fluid restrictions and perceived social support in patients receiving hemodialysis. Journal of Nursing Scholarship, 39(3), 243-248.

Karamanidou, C., Clatworthy, J., Weinman, J., & Horne, R. (2008). A systematic review of the prevalence and determinants of nonadherence to phosphate binding medication in patients with end-stage renal disease. [Comparative Study Research Support, Non-U.S. Gov't Review]. BMC Nephrology, 9, 2. doi: 10.1186/1471-2369-9-2

Karamanidou, C., Weinman, J., & Horne, R. (2008a). Improving haemodialysis patients' understanding of phosphate-binding medication: A pilot study of a psycho-educational intervention designed to change patients' perceptions of the problem and treatment. British journal of health psychology, 13, 205-214.

Kaveh, K., & Kimmel, P. L. (2001). Compliance in Hemodialysis Patients: Multidimensional Measures in Search of a Gold Standard. American Journal of Kidney Disease, 37(2), 244-266.

Khalil, A. A., & Frazier, S. K. (2010). Depressive symptoms and dietary nonadherence in patients with end-stage renal disease receiving hemodialysis: a review of quantitative evidence. [Research Support, N.I.H., Extramural Review]. Issues in mental health nursing, 31(5), 324-330. doi: 10.3109/01612840903384008

Khalil, A. A., Frazier, S. K., Lennie, T. A., & Sawaya, B. P. (2011). Depressive symptoms and dietary adherence in patients with end-stage renal disease. Journal of Renal Care, 37(1), 30-39.

Killingworth, A. (1993). Psychosocial impact of end-stage renal disease. British journal of nursing, 2(18), 905-908.

Kimmel, P. L., Peterson, R. A., Weihs, K. L., Simmens, S. J., Boyle, D. H., Verme, D., Cruz, I. (1995). Behavioral compliance with dialysis prescription in hemodialysis patients. Journal of the American Society of Nephrology, 5(10), 1826-1834.

Knobel H, Alonso J, Casado JL, Collazos J, Gonzalez J, et al., (2002) Validation of a simplified medication adherence questionnaire in a large cohort of HIV-infected patients: the GEEMA Study. AIDS 16, 605-613.

Kugler, C., Maeding, I., & Russel, C. L. (2011). Non-adherence in patients on chronic hemodialysis: an international comparison study. Journal of Nephrology, 24(3), 366-375.

Kugler, C., Vlaminck, H., Haverich, A., & Maes, B. (2005). Nonadherence With Diet and Fluid Restrictions Among Adults Having Hemodialysis. Journal of Nursing Scholarship, 37(1), 25-29.

Kutner, N. G., Zhang, R., McClellan, W. M., & Cole, S. A. (2002). Psychosocial predictors of non-compliance in haemodialysis and peritoneal dialysis patients. Nephro Dial Transplant, 17(1), 93-99.

Lam, L. W., Twinn, S. F., & Chan, S. W. C. (2010). Self-reported adherence to a therapeutic regimen among patients undergoing continuous ambulatory peritoneal dialysis. Journal of Advanced Nursing, 66(4), 763-773.

Lee, S. H., & Molassiotis, A. (2002). Dietary and fluid compliance in Chinese hemodialysis patients. Int J Nurs Stud, 39(7), 695-704.

Leggat, J. E., Jr. (2005). Adherence with dialysis: a focus on mortality risk. [Review]. Seminars in dialysis, 18(2), 137-141. doi: 10.1111/j.1525-139X.2005.18212.x

Leggat, J. E., Jr., Orzol, S. M., & Hulbert-Shearon, T. E., Golper T.A., Jones, C.A., Held, P.J. & Fort, F.K. (1998). Non-compliance in hemodialysis: Predictors and survival analysis. Am J Kidney Dis, 32(1), 139-145.

Lehane, E., & McCarthy, G. (2007). Intentional and unintentional medication non-adherence: a comprehensive framework for clinical research and practice? A discussion paper. International Journal of Nursing Studies, 44(8), 1468-1477.

Lin, C. C., & Liang, C. C. (1997). The relationship between health locus of control and compliance of hemodialysis patients. Kaohsiung J Med Sci, 13(4), 243-254.

Lindberg, M., Lindberg, P., & Wikstrom, B. (2007). Medication discrepancy: A concordance problem between dialysis patients and caregivers. Scandinavian journal of urology and nephrology, 41(6), 546-552.

Lindberg, M., Prutz, K., Lindberg, P., & Wikstrom, B. (2009). Interdialytic weight gain and ultrafiltration rate in hemodialysis: lessons about fluid adherence from a national registry of clinical practice. Hemodialysis International, 13(2), 181-188.

Lindquist, L. A., Go, L., Fleisher, J., Jain, N., Friesema, E., & Baker, D. W. (2012). Relationship of health literacy to intentional and unintentional non-adherence of hospital discharge medications. Journal of General Internal Medicine, 27(2), 173-178.

Loghman-Adhams, M. (2003). Medication noncompliance in patients with chronic disease: issues in dialysis and renal transplantation. Am J Manag Care, 9(2), 155-171.

Lopes, A. A., Bragg-Gresham, J. L., Satayathum, S., McCullough, K., Pifer, T., Goodkin, D. A., Port, F. K. (2003). Health-related quality of life and associated outcomes among hemodialysis patients of different ethnicities in the united states - the dialysis outcomes and practice patterns study (DOPPS). American Journal of Kidney Disease, 41(3), 605-615.

Lysaght, M. J. (2002). Maintenance Dialysis Population Dynamics: Current Trends and Long-Term Implications. Journal of the American Society of Nephrology, 13(Suppl 1), S37-S40.

Manley, H. J., Garvin, C. G., Drayer, D. K., Reid, G. M., Bender, W. L., Neufeld, T. K.,... Muther, R. S. (2004). Medication prescribing patterns in ambulatory haemodialysis patients: comparisons of USRDS to a large not-for-profit dialysis provider. Nephro Dial Transplant, 19(7), 1842-1848.

Mapes, D. L., Lopes, A. A., Satayathum, S., McCullough, K., Goodkin, D. A., Locatelli, F.,... Port, F. K. (2003). Health-related quality of life as a predictor of mortality and hospitalization: the dialysis outcomes and practice patterns study (DOPPS). Kidney Int, 64(1), 339-349.

Matteson, M. L., & Russell, C. (2010). Interventions to improve hemodialysis adherence: A systematic review of randomized-controlled trials. Hemodialysis International, 14(4), 370-382.

Morisky, D. E., Green, L. W., & Levine, D. M. (1986). Concurrent and predictive validity of a self-reported measure of medication adherence. Medical Care, 24(1), 67-74.

National Kidney Foundation. (2012). Dialysis. Retrieved 12 July, 2012, from http://www.kidney.org/atoz/content/dialysisinfo.cfm

Neri, L., Martini, A., Andreucci, V. E., Gallieni, M., Rey, L. A., Brancaccio, D., & MigliorDialisi Study Group. (2011). Regimen complexity and prescription adherence in dialysis patients. American journal of nephrology, 34(1), 71-76.

Rahman, M., & Griffin, V. (2004). Patterns of antihypertensive medication use in hemodialysis patients. American Journal of Health-system pharmacy, 61(14), 1473-1478.

Russell, C. L., Knowles, N., & Peace, L. (2007). Adherence in dialysis patients: a review of the literature. J Nephro Soc Work, 27, 11-44.

Sabate, E. (2003). Adherence to Long-Term Therapies: Evidence for Action. Geneva: World Health Organization.

Saran, R., Bragg-Gresham, J. L., & Rayner, H. C. (2003). Non-adherence in hemodialysis: Associations with mortality, hospitalization, and practice patterns in the DOPPS. Kidney Int, 64(254-262).

Schmid, H., Hartmann, B., & Schiffl, H. (2009). Adherence to Prescribed Oral Medication in Adult Patients Undergoing Chronic Hemodialysis: A Critical Review of the Literature. European Journal of Medical Research, 14(5), 185-190.

Segura-Orti, E., & Johansen, K. L. (2010). Exercise in end-stage renal disease. Seminars in dialysis, 23(4), 422-430.

Sharp, J., Wild, M. R., & Gumley, A. I. (2005). A Systematic Review of Psychological Interventions for the Treatment of Nonadherence to Fluid-Intake Restrictions in People Receiving Hemodialysis. Am J Kidney Dis, 45(1), 15-27.

Sharp, J., Wild, M. R., & Gumley, A. I. (2005a). A Cognitive Behavioral Group Approach to Enhance Adherence to Hemodialysis Fluid Restrictions: A Randomized Controlled Trial. American Journal of kidney Diseases, 45(6), 1046-1057.

Smart, N., & Steele, M. (2011). Exercise training in haemodialysis patients: a systematic review and meta-analysis. Nephrology (Carlton), 16(7), 626-632.

Sokol, M. C., McGuigan, K. A., Verbrugge, R. R., & Epstein, R. S. (2005). Impact of medication adherence on hospitalization risk and healthcare cost. Medical care, 43(6), 521-530.

Steenkamp, R., Castledine, C., Feest, T., & Fogarty, D. (2010). UK RRT Prevalence in 2009: national and centre-specific analyses The Thirteenth Annual Report (pp. 35-60). Bristol: The UK Renal Registry.

Sunanda, K., & Fadia, S. (2008). Medication non-adherence is associate with increased medical health care costs. Digestive diseases and sciences, 53(4), 1020-1024.

Theofilou, P. (2012). Medication adherence in Greek hemodialysis patients: the contribution of depression and health cognitions. International Journal of Behavioral Medicine, DOI 10.1007/s12529-012-9231-8.

Theofilou, P. (2012a). Results from the translation and cultural adaptation of the Greek Simplified Medication Adherence Questionnaire (GR-SMAQ) in patients with lung cancer. Journal of Clinical Trials, S:1, 1-3.

Tomasello, S., Dhupar, S., & Sherman, R. A. (2004). Phosphate binders, K/DOQI guidelines, and compliance: The unfortunate reality. Dialysis & transplantation, 33(5), 236-242.

Tracy, H. M., Green, C., & McCleary, J. (1987). Noncompliance in hemodialysis patients as measured with the MBHI. Psychology & health, 1(4), 411-423.

Tsay, S. L. (2003). Self-efficacy training for patients with end-stage renal disease. [Clinical Trial Randomized Controlled Trial Research Support, Non-U.S. Gov't]. Journal of Advanced Nursing, 43(4), 370-375.

U.S. Renal Data System. (2011). USRDS 2011 Annual Data Report: Atlas of Chronic Kidney Disease and End-Stage Renal Disease in the United States. In National Institutes of Health National Institute of Diabetes and Digestive and Kidney Diseases (Ed.). Bethesda MD,.

Unni, E. J., & Farris, K. B. (2011). Unintentional non-adherence and belief in medicines in older adults. Patient education and counseling, 83(2), 265-268.

Unruh, M. L., Evans, I. V., Fink, N. E., Powe, N. R., & Meyer, K. B. (2005). Skipped treatments, markers of nutritional nonadherence, and survival among incident hemodialysis patients. [Multicenter Study Research Support, N.I.H., Extramural Research Support, Non-U.S. Gov't Research Support, U.S. Gov't, P.H.S.]. American journal of kidney diseases: the official journal of the National Kidney Foundation, 46(6), 1107-1116. doi: 10.1053/j.ajkd.2005.09.002

Untas, A., Thumma, J., Rascle, N., Rayner, H., Mapes, D., Lopes, A. A., Combe, C. (2011). The associations of social support and other psychosocial factors with mortality and quality of life in the dialysis outcomes and practice patterns study. Clinical Journal of the American Society of Nephrology, 6(1), 142-152.

Valderrabano, F., Jofre, R., & Lopez-Gomez, J. M. (2001). Quality of life in end-stage renal disease patients. American Journal of Kidney Disease, 38(3), 443-464.

van Camp, Y. P., Huybrechts, S. A., van Rompaey, B., & Elseviers, M. M. (2011). Nurse-led education and counseling to enhance adherence to phosphate binders. Journal of clinical nursing, 21(9-10), 1304-1313.

van Dulmen, S., Sluijs, E., van Dijk, L., de Ridder, D., Heerdink, R., & Bensing, J. (2007). Patient adherence to medical treatment: a review of reviews. BMC health services research, 7(55).

Vlaminck, H., Maes, B., Jacobs, A., Reyntjens, S., & Evers, G. (2001). The Dialysis Diet and Fluid Non-adherence Questionnaire: validity testing of a self-report instrument for clinical practice. Journal of clinical nursing, 10(5), 707-715.

Weed-Collins, M., & Hogan, R. (1989). Knowledge and health beliefs regarding phosphate-binding medication in predicting compliance. ANNA journal / American Nephrology Nurses' Association, 16(4), 278-282.

Welch, J. L., & Thomas-Hawkins, C. (2005). Psycho-educational strategies to promote fluid adherence in adult hemodialysis patients: a review of intervention studies. Int J Nurs Stud, 42(5), 597-608.

Wells, J. R. (2011). Hemodialysis knowledge and medical adherence in African Americans diagnosed with end stage renal disease: results of an educational intervention. [Research Support, Non-U.S. Gov't Review]. Nephrology nursing journal : journal of the American Nephrology Nurses' Association, 38(2), 155-162; quiz 163.

Wroe, A. L. (2002). Intentional and unintentional nonadherence: a study of decision making. Journal of behavioral medicine, 25(4), 355-372.

Send Orders of Reprints at reprints@benthamscience.net

CHAPTER 8

A Systematic Review of Interventions to Increase Hemodialysis Adherence: 2007-2012

Michelle L. Matteson[1,*] and Cynthia Russell[2]

[1]*Department of Gastroenterology and Hepatology, University of Missouri, USA and* [2]*University of Missouri-Kansas City, School of Nursing, USA*

Abstract: Hemodialysis involves a complex regimen involving adherence to treatment, fluid, medication and diet prescriptions. Studies examining adherence to treatment, fluid, medication and diet prescriptions in adult hemodialysis patients from 2007 to May 2012 were reviewed and results presented. Eleven studies (two randomized controlled trial and nine quasi-experimental studies) were identified attempting to enhance hemodialysis adherence. A randomized controlled trial study design with a large, diverse nonadherent sample testing a theory-based intervention delivered by multi-disciplinary teams address the system in which the patient functions may enhance adherence to treatment, fluid, medication and diet adherence.

Keywords: Hemodialysis, adherence, diet, fluid, interventions, dialysis treatment, systematic review, adult, nonadherence, efficacy, IDWG, hyperphosphatemia, hypoalbuminemia, missed treatments, shortened treatments, treatment adequacy, cognitive intervention, behavioral intervention, affective intervention, personal system-focused intervention.

INTRODUCTION

Over 870,000 people in the United States are being treated for end-stage kidney disease, and almost 400,000 of those are receiving dialysis (United States Renal Data System [USRDS], 2011). In 2009, $82,285 was spent on each hemodialysis patient receiving Medicare in the United States (USRDS).

As the number of hemodialysis patients continues to increase, identifying successful adherence interventions is vital to the health of this population. The purpose of this chapter is to update our previously published systematic review of interventions to increase treatment, fluid, medication and diet adherence in adult hemodialysis patients (Matteson, & Russell, 2010). This systematic review will include both randomized controlled trials and quasi-experimental study designs.

*Address correspondence to Michelle L. Matteson: Department of Gastroenterology/Hepatology, University of Missouri, Columbia, MO, USA; Tel: 573-289-2098; Fax: 573-884-8200; E-mail: mattesonml@health.missouri.edu

Paraskevi Theofilou (Ed)

Hemodialysis involves complicated treatment prescriptions. Adherence, defined by the World Health Organization, is "the extent to which a person's behavior (taking medications, following a recommended diet, and/or executing lifestyle changes) corresponds with the agreed recommendations of a health care provider" (Sabate, 2003, p. 13). Complex and long-term treatment can contribute to nonadherence (McDonald, Garg, & Haynes, 2002); thus nonadherence to hemodialysis treatment is high as it requires three times a week hemodialysis, diet and fluid restrictions, and medication adherence. Typical patients are prescribed 10 or more medications per day. Nonadherence measures have been published by the National Kidney Foundation to standardize outcomes and quality indicators. The Kidney Dialysis Outcome and Quality Initiative (KDOQI) guidelines document the nonadherence levels for missed or shortened treatments, inter-dialytic weight gain (IDWG), serum phosphorus, serum albumin, and treatment adequacy (Kt/V) (Saran *et al.*, 2003) (Table **1**).

Table 1: KDOQI guidelines-Nonadherence measures (Kt/V=measure of dialysis adequacy; kg/day=killigrams per day; mg/dl=milligrams per deciliter; g/dL=grams per deciliter).

Missed treatment	**Attendance at less than the prescribed number of weekly dialysis treatments**
Shortened treatments	Shortening a single prescribed dialysis treatment by 10 minutes or greater
Interdialytic Weight Gain (IDWG)	<1.0kg/day
Serum Phosphorous	<3.5 or >5.5mg/dL
Kt/V	<1.2
Serum Albumin	<4.0 g/dL

Dialysis treatment, medication, and diet nonadherence rates are unacceptably high (Russell, *et al.*, 2008). In a recent study, overall diet nonadherence was 80.4% and fluid nonadherence 75.3% (Kugler, Maeding, & Russell, 2011). In a study by Kim and Evangelista (2010), nonadherence to missed and/or shortened hemodialysis treatments was 12.6%, followed by nonadherence to fluid restrictions 20.5%, and medication and diet 31.8%. When examined alone, medication nonadherence rates in dialysis patients ranged from 3-80% (Karamanidou, Clatworthy, Weinman & Horne, 2008). Specifically, nonadherence to phosphate binding medication in adult peritoneal and hemodialysis patients ranged from 22-74% with a mean of

51% (Karamanidou, Clatworthy, Weinman, & Horne, 2008). Hemodialysis nonadherence rates are suboptimal.

Hemodialysis nonadherence results in higher rates of morbidity, hospitalization and mortality (Leggat *et al.*, 1998; Obialo, 2012; Saran *et al.*, 2003). Missed and shortened treatments can increase risk for cardiovascular events (Leggat *et al.*, 1998; Saran *et al.*, 2003). Nonadherence to medications and diet can result in hyperphosphatemia which has been found to increase cardiovascular disease and fracture risk (Block *et al.*, 2004).

Interventions to enhance health behaviors have been classified into four areas: cognitive, behavioral, affective, and personal system-focused. Cognitive interventions aim to increase patients' knowledge of their disease or medications (Peterson, Takiya, & Finley, 2003). Behavioral interventions involve changing health behaviors through motivation and intention, whereas affective interventions strive to change attitudes, values and beliefs (Peterson, Takiya, & Finley, 2003). Personal system-based interventions identify personal system changes through a process of Plan-Do-Check-Act (Russell, 2010).

METHODS

The Cumulative Index of Nursing and Allied Health Literature (CINAHL) (2007 to May 2012), MEDLINE (2007 to May 2012), PsychINFO (2007 to May 2012), and all Evidence-Based Medicine (EBM) Reviews (Cochran DSR, ACP Journal Club, DARE, and CCTR) were searched to identify studies testing efficacy of interventions to improve adherence to treatment, fluid, medication and diet adherence in adult hemodialysis patients from 2007 to May 2012. The search terms used were as follows: dialysis, hemodialysis, haemodialysis, kidney failure, kidney, articial, intervention, complian*, noncomplian*, non-complian* adheren*, nonadheren*, non-adheren*, concordance, non-concordance, medication, drugs, and diet*, or fluid* or nutrition* or phosphate* or drinking were used. Inclusion criteria for study design were a randomized controlled trial or quasi-experimental design (lacking randomization and/or a control group) testing an intervention directed at increasing adherence to treatment, fluid, medication and diet adherence in adult hemodialysis patients. The RCT is considered the strongest study design

(Polit, & Beck, 2012), but due to the limited number of RCT's since our last review, quasi-experimental studies were included for this review. Data were extracted from peer-reviewed studies by the authors (MM and CR). Data extraction included author and year, sample/setting, study design, intervention description (dose and duration), theory, measures, results, strengths and weaknesses and are noted in Table **2**. As with our previous review, CONSORT and STROBE guidelines were used to evaluate the strength of the study reporting details (Matteson, & Russell, 2010).

Measures

In order to score methodological quality of the included studies, CONSORT and STROBE reporting guidelines were utilized. The CONSORT criteria were used to evaluate the quality of the methodologic reporting details of the two randomized controlled trials (Morey *et al.*, 2008; de Araujo *et al.*, 2010). CONSORT scores can range from 0-22, with 22 reflecting high quality study detail reporting (Schulz, Altman, & Moher, 2010). CONSORT scores for the articles are found in Table **3**.

The STROBE criteria were used to score the quality of the methodologic reporting of the nine quasi-experimental studies (Baraz, 3009; Best, 2011; Gardulf, 2011; Kandiah, 2010; Katzir *et al.*, 2010; Russell *et al.*, 2011; Satoh, 2009; Van Camp, 2011; Wells, 2011). STROBE scores can range from 0-22. A STROBE score of 22 indicates a highest quality of reporting observational study details (von Elm *et al.*, 2007). The eleven studies were scored by the reviewers and scores were agreed upon. Table **4** reflects the STROBE scoring details.

Table 2: Hemodialysis pre-post studies reviewed. Abbreviations: Hemodialysis (HD); Continuous Ambulatory Peritoneal Dialysis (CAPD); average (x); intervention (I); control (C); Time on Dialysis (TOD); primary investigator (PI); randomized control trial (RCT); Quality of Life=QOL; medication electronic monitoring system (MEMS); not recorded (NR).

Author/Design	Purpose	Sample/Setting	Intervention	Intervention type	Measures	Results	Strengths/limitations
Morey, Walker, & Davenport (2008) RCT	Determine effect of monthly dietetic consultations on patient's serum phosphate concentrations and calcium x phosphate product	N=67 HD patients with hyperphosphatemia Age x (I)=60.4 years Age x (C)=54.9 years TOD x (I)= 45 months (range 7-327) TOD x (C)=41 months (range 6-283) Country: United Kingdom	Interventionist: Dietitian Description: Individualized, strategies include motivational counseling, negotiation, behavior modification therapy, reminders, reinforcement, supportive care and both written and verbal education aimed at limiting phosphorus dietary intake and increasing compliance with phosphate binders Dose: Monthly for 6 months Duration: 6 months Follow up: NR	Cognitive-behavioral	Serum phosphorus Self-report Adherence	Within intervention group, serum phosphate level decreased at 3 months (p=0.0030), but no statistical difference noted at 6 months; no statistically significant change in calcium x phosphate product Within control group, no statistically significant difference in serum phosphorous level noted; statistically significant decrease in calcium x phosphate product (p=0.048) Between groups: No statistically significant difference in serum phosphorus levels at 6 or 12 months Statistically significant decrease in the calcium	Strengths: Nonadherent participants defined as those with hyperphosphatemia Strong design PI blinded to group assignment Limitations: No theoretical basis Self-reported adherence measure Underpowered to detect group differences

Table 2: contd....

De Araujo, Figueiredo, d'Avila (2010) RCT	Determine effect of educational program on adherence	N=33 (I)n=16; © n=17 Description: Age x=52.5 years Men n=18 (55%) TOD x=19.9 months (range 7.8-38 months) Country: Brazil Calcium, phosphorus, and parathyroid metabolism education to 1 group; ©group given information on vascular access, types of catheters, and arteriovenous graft Dose: 30 minutes Duration: 3 months Follow-up: 30, 60, 90 days	Interventionist: NR	Calcium, phosphorus, BUN, Creatinine, and parathyroid hormone at the beginning of each month; Kt/V	No statistically significant results between groups. All biochemical exams improved but not statistically significant within the groups and no between group statistically significant results were found. No statistically significant results between groups; All biochemical exams improved but not statistically significant within the groups and no between group statistically significant results were found. No differences in self-reported patient compliance within groups or between groups x phosphate product at 3 months (p<0.05)	Strengths: RCT Limitations: Small sample Eight patients left study (2 quit; 2 transplanted; 4 left to other motives) No theoretical basis
Russell, Cronk, Herron, Knowles, Matteson, Peace, & Ponferrada (2011)	To examine the feasibility and efficacy of a staff-delivered motivational interviewing technique on	N=29 outpatient HD patients Female 53% (n=10) Caucasian 68% (n=13) Description:	Interventionist: Dialysis nurses/staff (technicians, dietitian, social worker) Description: Cognitive-behavioral	Dialysis attendance, frequency of shortened treatments, phosphorous, albumin, IDWG,	MI positively affected missed treatments-5 (26%) improved, 13 (68%) unchanged 1 (6%) worsened; shortened treatments- 9 (47%) improved, 6	Strengths: Intervention delivered by nurses and dialysis staff with fidelity checks

Table 2: contd....

Citation / Design	Purpose	Sample / Country	Intervention	Theory	Measures	Results	Strengths / Weaknesses
Pilot Pre-Post design	treatment, diet, medication, and fluid adherence	Country: US	Motivational interviewing (MI) is client-centered, semi-directive method of tapping into the individual's motivation to change behavior by developing discrepancy between current and ideal functioning, and exploring the resolving ambivalence within the individual. Dose: every dialysis session. Dose: Every dialysis session (3 times per week). Duration: 3 months. Follow-up: 3 months	Cognitive	Health Care Climate Questionnaire (HCCQ) scores	(27%) unchanged, 4 (27%) worsened; dietary phosphorus- 6 (32%) improved, 9 (47%) unchanged, 4 (21%) worsened; and albumin levels- 4 (21%) improved, 14 (73%) unchanged, 1 (6%) worsened. MI less favorable change with IDWG- 2 (11.1%) improved, 12 (63%) unchanged, 5 (26%) worsened. Changes in HCCQ questionnaire not statistically significant ($p=0.15$) but in anticipated duration for autonomy support	Weaknesses: Pre-post design. Pilot study. Small sample. No theoretical basis
Katzir, Boaz, Backshi, Cernes, Barnea & Biro (2010). Pre-post design	Determine the effect of an education program on medication compliance and knowledge	N=89 (75 HD; 14 CAPD). Age x=62.7 years. Female=34. TOD x=5 years +/- 4.25 years	Interventionist: nephrologist. Description: Oral/written instructions (drug information manuals were orally explained and distributed to		Self report education of medication adherence and medication knowledge of five groups of medications	Self report compliance increased from 89 to 95.7 % ($p=0.0007$) with compliance increases in HD more than CAPD ($p=0.0001$). Increased Calcium ($p=0.0001$)	Strengths: 3 months follow-up. Weaknesses: Pre-post design. Small sample size

Table 2: contd....

Author / Study	Purpose	Sample	Intervention	Theory	Labs / Measures	Results	Strengths / Limitations
		Country: Israel (each participant)	The information in the manual was reviewed 3 months later. Dose: 2 doses 3 months apart. Duration: 3 months. Follow-up: 6 months	Cognitive-behavioral	Labs pre and post: serum calcium, phosphorus, parathyroid, hemoglobin, hematocrit and mcv	Decreased parathyroid (p=0.006). Decreased potassium (p=0.02). Decreased phosphorus (p=0.06). Decreased IDWG (p=0.07)	No theoretical basis
Kandiah, Resler, & Amend (2010) Pilot pre-post study	Evaluate the effectiveness of a nutritional theme game "National Fosphorus League Phootball'	N=66 HD patients. Males 50%. Age range= 18-76. TOD 1-3 years (35%). Country: US	Interventionist: Dietitian. Description: Nutrition education handouts and several motivational tools/handouts (1-1 counseling, handouts and quiz). Dose: monthly (time not documented). Duration: 4 months. Follow-up: 6 months	Cognitive-behavioral	Serum phosphorus and calcium-phosphorus product baseline and end of 4 month intervention	No statistically significant results; however, improvement in phosphorus and calcium-phosphorus were noted. Six months after end of study these levels were decreased, but not statistically significant	Strengths: 6 month follow-up. Limitations: Small sample. No statistically significant results. No theoretical basis
Gardulf, Palsson, & Nicolay (2011) Pre-post study	Determining the effects of an educational program on biological, knowledge,	N=43 HD nonadherent to phosphate binders based on serum levels	Interventionist: educational team consisting of 1-2 RN(s), a dietitian and a nephrologist)	Cognitive-behavioral	Knowledge (pre-post); self-report Phosphate, albumin,	Statistically significant increase in knowledge (p=0.001). Phosphate, albumin, Statistically significant	Strengths: Nonadherent participants. Mean serum phosphorus level at baseline was within the KDOQI target range. No theoretical basis

Table 2: contd.....

Citation	Purpose	Sample	Description	Interventionist / Type	Measures	Results	Strengths / Limitations
	behavioral and health related quality of life (QOL) of self-dosing of phosphate binders	Men n=34 Age x=60.7 years (range 30-82) TOD: 31 months (range 1-152 months) Country: Sweden	Description: Structured educational program regarding calcium and phosphate balance, food intake and phosphate binders (session 1- meet/greet activities; session 2/3 targeted to learn calcium and phosphate balance, symptoms and complications of high phosphorus; session 4/5 focused on self-care) Dose: 60 minutes 3-5 times (group discussions) Duration: 2 months Follow-up: 12 months		corrected calcium, intact parathyroid hormone levels (pre-post, 3, 6, 9, 12 months after the end of the educational program) Health related quality of life (HRQL) and short-Form 36 (SF-36) Food diary	decrease in phosphate level at 2 months (p=0.05) and at 12 months (p=0.001)	12 month study follow-up Limitations: Self-report of knowledge and QOL Small sample 25% of sample lost to follow-up and not given the study specific questionnaire Study specific questionnaire (knowledge of calcium/phosphorus balance and HRQL) has had no validity or reliability testing performed No theoretical basis
Best, Canny, Averette, Cameron, Keaveney, Anderson, Stroman, Felts, Lapinski, Grammas, & Russ (2011)	Effect of focused patient education and individualized social work interventions on missed HD treatments	N=219 non adherent HD patients(non-adherence based on missed treatments in those with mental health problems) Country: US	Interventionist: social workers Description: Education regarding the impact of patient nonadherence on health and	Cognitive-behavioral	Missed treatments	Missed treatments reduced or eliminated in 71% of patients Overall missed treatment reschedule rate doubled from 0.35% in July 2007 to 0.68% in June 2008	Strengths: Nonadherent sample Limitations: Abstract only (study details are limited) Pre-post design

Table 2: contd....

Citation/Design	Purpose	Sample	Intervention	Theory	Measures	Results	Strengths/Weaknesses
Pre-post			interventions such as teaching relaxation techniques, providing direction for substance abuse treatment or solving scheduling issues; a 'social work intervention' Dose: individualized based on need Duration: 12 months Follow-up: Not reported			Combined missed treatment rate for non-adherence was 1.77% compared to baseline rate of 4.22% in July 2007.	No theoretical basis Sample size unknown
Satoh, Koizumi, Izumi, Kugoh, Kiriyama,... & Hirata (2009) Pre/post design	Investigate the effectiveness of a pharmacist- provided education regarding phosphate binders and hyperphosphatemia on serum phosphate concentration and calcium and calcium x phosphorus product	N=398 HD patients Age: NR TOD: NR Country: Japan	Interventionist: Pharmacist Description: Individualized education based on baseline knowledge questionnaire; the more nonadherent the more education was given; pharmacist discussed 3 points: hyper- phosphatemia, taking phosphate binders, and carrying binders with them at all times. Dose: 1 time	Cognitive	Serum phosphorus, calcium, BUN, creatinine, albumin and hemoglobin averaged two months before the intervention and two months after the intervention	Statistically significant decrease in both serum phosphorus > 7.0mg/dL and calcium/phosphate product (p<0.001). Statistically significant decrease in phosphorus (6.0-6.9mg/dL) (p<0.05) and calcium/phosphate product (p<0.005)	Strengths: Large sample size. Weakness: No theoretical basis Pre-post design Intervention directed at all participants but authors stratified the adherence levels to determine effect.

Table 2: contd....

| Wells (2011) Three-group quasi experimental design | Describe the relationship between hemodialysis knowledge and perceived medication adherence; determine if an educational intervention improved HD knowledge and medical adherence | N=85 African American HD patients (Group 1 n=27; Group 2 n=29; Group 3 n=29) Options Age X=52.5 years (range 20-86) TOD: 66% 1-5 years Female n= 45 (52.9%) Country: US | Duration: 20-40 minutes Follow up: None Interventionist: PhD-prepared nurse One-on-one session based on principles related to ESRD and HD based on the Life Options Hemodialysis Knowledge Test and content received by patients from the HD interdisciplinary teams (kidney function, dietary and fluid restrictions, lab values and medications associated with ESRD, HD process and adherence to treatment regimen Group 1: pretest, educational intervention, handout of content, and posttest; Group 2: pretest, no educational intervention, a | Cognitive | Life Options Hemodialysis Knowledge Test; Medical Outcomes Study (MOS) | Group 1: statistically significant difference in knowledge found within group I (p<0.01; 95% CI=-4.51 to -1.34) No statistically significant difference in medication adherence (based on MOS scores) within group I (p>0.01) No group 2 or group 3 were statistically significant and may have had health literacy issues No significant correlational relationship found between HD knowledge and perceived medical adherence (pre-test and post-test p=0.78; post-test p=0.38) across the entire sample | Strengths: Three group design with control group Weaknesses: Quasi-experimental design (not randomized to groups) Lack of generalizability (all African American sample and lack of random sampling technique) Fidelity to the intervention Possible poor health literacy of the sample Small samples No theoretical basis Not fully powered study |

Table 2: contd....

| Baraz, Parvardeh, Mohammadi, & Broumand (2009)

Quasi-experimental design | Determine the effect of an educational intervention on dietary and fluid compliance | N=63 HD patients

Males n=33 (52.4%)

Age X=34.8 (range 18–50)

TOD: X=4.6 years (range 0.5–8 years)

Nonadherent=23 (based on IDWG)

Country: Iran | Interventionist: renal nurse expert

Description:

Group 1 (verbal education in group session): group education was interactive and didactic; encouraged to offer support to each other and received a teaching booklet to take home, "A Patient Guide to Controlling Dietary Regimen".

Group 2 (video education): individually approached during two consecutive dialysis session in a week; video shown to | Cognitive | Phosphate, calcium, sodium, potassium, uric acid, creatinine, albumin, BUN, and IDWG | Within groups:

Group 1: Statistically significant decreases noted in creatinine, phosphate, BUN and uric acid level.

Group 2: Statistically significant decrease in phosphate and uric acid level

Statistically significant increase in calcium levels

Between groups: No statistically significant difference in any biochemical parameter between the two educational interventions | Strengths:

Quasi-experimental design (with no control group)

Limitations:

Limited follow-up of 2 months

No long-term follow-up

No theoretical basis

2/3 of patients compliant at baseline |
| | | | handout of content taught, posttest;

Group 3: pretest and post-test only

Dose: 1 time

Duration: 30 minutes

Follow-up: 1 month | | | | |

Table 2: contd....

					each patient after 1-2 hours after initiation of HD (duration of the video-30 minutes).		
					Both groups: general knowledge about ESRD, dietary management for HD, identification of restricted/non-restricted food, fluid restrictions, reasons for compliance and possible consequences of noncompliance		Cognitive intervention increases the fluid and dietary compliance of HD patients (creatinine p=0.000); potassium p=0.018; calcium p=0.000; phosphate p=0.000; uric acid p=0.000; BUN p=0.000; IDWG p=0.000).
					Dose: 1 time		
					Duration: 30 minutes		
					Follow-up: 2 months		
Van Camp, Huybrechts, Van Rompaey, & Elseviers (2011)	Investigate nurse-led education and counseling enhance phosphate binder adherence	N=257(1 n=41;n=216 historical control group)	Interventionist: BSN nurse	Cognitive-behavioral	Adherence to phosphate binders was electronically monitored by MEMS; pill count and self-report of phosphate binders were used to corroborate the MEMS data.	Statistically significant decrease within the intervention group in phosphorus (p,0.001); calcium (p=0.002); knowledge (p<0.001)	Strengths: MEMS monitoring of phosphate binder adherence
Two groups (intervention and historical control)		Men 71%	Description: educational pamphlet and personalized counseling			Adherence increased from 82.5% to 94.4% in the(I) group and decreased in the historical © group	Study nurse, patient and site personnel blinded to adherence results
		Age range 40-83 age x=68	Dose:				
		Dialysis treatment period x=49 months	Educational session 1 time at week 5				Limitations:

Table 2: contd....

(range 4–267 months)			
Country: Belgium and Dutch dialysis centers	Counseling sessions lasted 20 minutes and delivered bi-weekly at weeks 7, 9, 11, 13, 15.	Secondary outcomes: serum phosphate, calcium, parathyroid hormone (PTH) and knowledge of phosphate binders. Phosphate and calcium collected weekly; PTH measure beginning and end of study. Knowledge assessed by 10 item multiple choice test.	85.5% to 75.9%	Historical control group Unequal time monitoring of MEMES (intervention group 17 weeks; control group 14 weeks) No theoretical basis No long term outcomes
	Duration: 17 weeks			
	Follow-up: Not reported			

Table 3: CONSORT scoring (0=not documented; 0.5 partially documented; 1=documented).

		Morey 2008	De Araujo 2010
	Title & abstract		
1	How participants were allocated to interventions (*e.g.,*, random allocation, randomized or randomly assigned)	1	0
	Introduction		
2	Background	Scientific background and explanation of rationale	1	0.5
	Methods		
3	Participants	Eligibility criteria for participants and the settings and locations where the data were collected	1	1

Table 3: contd....

4	Interventions	Precise details of the interventions intended for each group and how and when they were actually administered	1	0.5	
5	Objectives	Specific objectives and hypotheses	0.5	0.5	
6	Outcomes	Clearly defined primary and secondary outcome measures and, when applicable, any methods used to enhance the quality of measurements (*e.g.*, Multiple observations, training of assessors)	1	0.5	
7	Sample Size	How sample size was determined and, when applicable, explanation of any interim analyses and stopping rules	1	0.5	
Randomization					
8	Sequence generation	Method used to generate the random allocation sequence, including details of any restriction (*e.g.*, blocking, stratification)	1	0	
9	Allocation concealment	Method used to implement the random allocation sequence (*e.g.*, Numbered containers or central telephone), clarifying whether the sequence was concealed until interventions were assigned	0.5	0	
10	Implementation	Who generated the allocation sequence, who enrolled participants, and who assigned participants to their groups	0.5	0	
11	Blinding (masking)	Whether or not participants, those administrating the interventions, and those assessing the outcomes were blinded to group assignment. If done, how the success of blinding was evaluated	0.5	0	
12	Statistical methods	Statistical methods used to compare groups for primary outcome(s); methods for additional analyses, such as subgroup analyses and adjusted analyses.	1	1	
Results					
13	Participant flow	Flow of participants through each stage (a diagram is strongly recommended). Specifically, for each group report the numbers of participants randomly assigned, receiving intended treatment, completing the study protocol, and analyzed for the primary outcome. Describe protocol deviations from study as planned, together with reasons.	1	0	
14	Recruitment	Dates defining the periods of recruitment and follow-up.	1	0	
15	Baseline data	Baseline demographic and clinical characteristics of each group.	1	1	

Table 3: contd...

		Recommendation	Russell 2011	Sotah 2011
16	Numbers analyzed	Number of participants (denominator) in each group included in each analysis and whether the analysis was by intention to treat. State the results in absolute numbers when feasible (*e.g.,* 10/20, not 50%)	0.5	1
17	Outcomes and estimation	For each primary and secondary outcome, a summary of results for each group, and the estimated effect size and its precision (*e.g.,* 95% confidence interval)	0.5	0.5
18	Ancillary analyses	Address multiplicity by reporting any other analyses performed, including subgroup analyses and adjusted analyses, indicating those pre-specified and those exploratory.	0	0
19	Adverse events	All important adverse events of side effects in each intervention group	1	0.5
Discussion				
20	Interpretation	Interpretation of the results, taking into account study hypotheses; sources of potential bias or imprecision and the dangers associated with multiplicity of analyses and outcomes	1	1
21	Generalizability	Generalizability (external validity) of the trial findings	0.5	0.5
22	Overall evidence	General interpretation of the results in the context of current evidence	1	1
	Total score		17.5	10

Table 4: STROBE scoring (0=not documented; 0.5= partially documented; 1=documented).

	Item No	Recommendation	Russell 2011	Katzir 2010	Kandiah 2010	Gardulf 2011	Best 2011	Wells 2011	Baraz 2009	VanCamp 2011	Sotah 2011
Title and abstract	1	(*a*) Indicate the study's design with a commonly used term in the title or the abstract	0.5	0.5	0.5	0.5	0.5	0.5	0.5	0.5	0.5
		(*b*) Provide in the abstract an informative and balanced summary of what was done and what was found	0.5	0.5	0	0	0	0.5	0	0	0
Introduction Background/rationale	2	Explain the scientific background and rationale for the investigation being reported	1	1	1	1	0	1	1	1	1

Table 4: contd...

Objectives	3	State specific objectives, including any pre-specified hypotheses	1	1	1	1	1	1	1	0.5
Study design	4	Present key elements of study design early in the paper	1	1	1	1	1	0	1	0.5
Setting	5	Describe the setting, locations, and relevant dates, including periods of recruitment, exposure, follow-up, and data collection	1	0.5	1	0.5	0.5	0.5	1	1
Participants	6	*Case-control study*—Give the eligibility criteria, and the sources and methods of case ascertainment and control selection. Give the rationale for the choice of cases and controls	n/a	n/a	n/a	0.5	0.5	n/a	n/a	n/a
Variables	7	Clearly define all outcomes, exposures, predictors, potential confounders, and effect modifiers. Give diagnostic criteria, if applicable	1	1	1	1	0.5	1	1	1
Data sources/ measurement	8	For each variable of interest, give sources of data and details of methods of assessment (measurement). Describe comparability of assessment methods if there is more than one group	1	1	1	1	0	1	1	1
Bias	9	Describe any efforts to address potential sources of bias	0	0	0	0	0	0	1	0
Study size	10	Explain how the study size was arrived at	0	0	0	0	0	0	1	1
Quantitative variables	11	Explain how quantitative variables were handled in the analyses. If applicable, describe which groupings were chosen and why	1	1	1	1	0	1	1	1
Statistical methods	12	(*a*) Describe all statistical methods, including those used to control for confounding	1	1	0.5	1	1	1	1	1
		(*b*) Describe any methods used to examine subgroups and interactions	n/a	n/a	n/a	n/a	n/a	n/a	0	0
		(*c*) Explain how missing data were addressed	0	0	0	0	0	0	0	0
		(*d*) *Case-control study*—If applicable, explain how matching of cases and controls was addressed	n/a	n/a	n/a	n/a	n/a	n/a	n/a	n/a
		(*e*) Describe any sensitivity analyses	0	0	0	0	0	0	0	0
RESULTS Participants	13	(*a*) Report numbers of individuals at each stage of study—e.g., numbers potentially eligible, examined for eligibility, confirmed eligible, included in the study, completing follow-up, and analyzed	0.33	0	0	0.33	0	0	0	0.33
		(*b*) Give reasons for non-participation at each stage	0.33	0	0.33	0.33	0.33	n/a	0.33	0.33
		(*c*) Consider use of a flow diagram	0.33	0	0	0	0	0	0	0

Table 4: contd…

Descriptive data		Description									
Descriptive data	14	(a) Give characteristics of study participants (*e.g.*, demographic, clinical, social) and information on exposures and potential confounders	1	1	1	1	0	1	1	1	1
		(b) Indicate number of participants with missing data for each variable of interest	0	0	0	0	0	0	0	0	0
Outcome data	15	*Case-control study*—Report numbers in each exposure category, or summary measures of exposure	n/a	n/a	n/a	n/a	n/a	n/a	n/a	n/a	n/a
Main results	16	(*a*) Give unadjusted estimates and, if applicable, confounder-adjusted estimates and their precision (*e.g.*, 95% confidence interval). Make clear which confounders were adjusted for and why they were included	n/a	n/a	n/a	n/a	n/a	n/a	n/a	1	n/a
		(*b*) Report category boundaries when continuous variables were categorized	1	n/a	n/a	n/a	n/a	n/a	n/a	n/a	1
		(*c*) If relevant, consider translating estimates of relative risk into absolute risk for a meaningful time period	n/a	n/a	n/a	n/a	n/a	n/a	n/a	n/a	n/a
Other analyses	17	Report other analyses done—*e.g.*, analyses of subgroups and interactions, and sensitivity analyses	0	1	0	1	0	0	0	0	1
Key results	18	Summarizes key results with reference to study objectives	1	1	1	1	1	1	1	1	1
Limitations	19	Discuss limitations of the study, taking into account sources of potential bias or imprecision. Discuss both direction and magnitude of any potential bias	1	0.5	1	1	0	1	1	1	1
Interpretation	20	Give a cautious overall interpretation of results considering objectives, limitations, multiplicity of analyses, results from similar studies, and other relevant evidence	1	1	1	1	0.5	1	1	1	1
Generalizability	21	Discuss the generalizability (external validity) of the study results	1	0.5	0.5	1	0	1	1	1	1
Funding	22	Give the source of funding and the role of the funders for the present study and, if applicable, for the original study on which the present article is based	1	0	0	1	0	1	1	0	0
Totals	22		18	13.5	12.5	15.66	3.5	14.5	15.5	19.5	15.83

RESULTS

Eleven studies were identified and met inclusion criteria. Study designs ranged from two randomized control trials (RCT) (Morey *et al.*, 2008; de Araujo *et al.*, 2010) to nine quasi-experimental studies (Baraz, 3009; Best, 2011; Gardulf, 2011; Kandiah, 2010; Katzir *et al.*, 2010; Russell *et al.*, 2011; Satoh, 2009; Van Camp, 2011; Wells, 2011). Sample sizes ranged from 29 (Russell *et al.*, 2011) to 398 (Satoh, 2009). Nonadherent samples were the focus of three of the studies (Morey *et al.*, 2008; Gardulf *et al.*, 2011; Best *et al.*, 2011).

The setting of the studies varied greatly; four of the eleven studies were from the United States (Russell *et al.*, 2011; Kandiah, Resler & Amend, 2010; Best *et al.*, 2011; Wells, 2011) with the remaining studies from Belgium (VanCamp *et al.*, 2011), Brazil (de Araujo, Figueiredo, d'Avila, 2010), Japan (Satoh *et al.*, 2009), Iran (Baraz *et al.*, 2009), Israel (Katzir *et al.*, 2010), Sweden (Gardulf, Palsson & Nicolay, 2011), and the United Kingdom (Morey *et al.*, 2008).

The strength of the reporting details was evaluated by the CONSORT and STROBE criteria. Two randomized controlled trials were evaluated based on the CONSORT criteria. The CONSORT scoring ranged from 10 (de Araujo, 2010) to 17.5 (Morey, 2008). Nine quasi-experimental studies were scored *via* the STROBE criteria (Baraz, 3009; Best, 2011; Gardulf, 2011; Kandiah, 2010; Katzir *et al.*, 2010; Russell *et al.*, 2011; Satoh, 2009; Van Camp, 2011; Wells, 2011). The STROBE scoring ranged from 3 (Best *et al.*, 2011) to 19.5 (Van Camp *et al.*, 2011).

The interventions utilized in the eleven studies can be classified into two categories: cognitive interventions (Baraz, 3009; de Araujo, 2010; Katzir *et al.*, 2010; Satoh, 2009; Wells, 2011), and cognitive-behavioral interventions (Best, 2011; Gardulf, 2011; Kandiah, 2010; Morey, 2008; Russell *et al.*, 2011; Van Camp, 2011). There were no affective or personal system-focused interventions tested.

Five cognitive interventions were directed towards improving medication, diet and fluid adherence. Two studies targeted medication nonadherence (phosphate binder) where as three studies targeted diet and fluid nonadherence. Katzir *et al.,* (2010) and Satoh *et al.,* (2009) targeted individualized phosphate binder education based on results of questionnaires. Baraz *et al.,* (2009) focused a cognitive intervention on dietary and fluid adherence *via* oral/video instruction in a group format. DeAraujo *et al.,* (2010) tested a calcium, phosphorus, and parathyroid metabolism education program aimed at decreasing nonadherence. Wells (2011) used education regarding dietary and fluid restrictions, lab values and medications based on pretest information from the Life Options Hemodialysis Knowledge Test to enhance adherence.

The six cognitive-behavioral interventions focused on motivation and intention to improve adherence through disease/medication education and self-care/management. Russell and colleagues (2011) trained dialysis staff to use motivational interviewing to improve treatment, fluid, and diet adherence (Russell *et al.*, 2011). Two other studies used motivational counseling/tools and education to increase adherence to phosphate binders (Morey, Walker, & Davenport, 2008; Kandiah, Resler & Amend, 2010). Gardulf and colleagues addressed phosphate binder adherence through a structured educational program with self-care sessions (Gardulf, Palsson, & Nicolay, 2011). Best and colleagues used a 'social work intervention' focusing on the effects of nonadherence on health, and teaching interventions such as relaxation techniques or help with dialysis scheduling issues (Best *et al.*, 2011). Finally, a sixth study used an educational pamphlet and personalized counseling to enhance phosphate binder adherence (Van Camp *et al.*, 2011). No studies utilized a theoretical basis for the intervention.

The dose of the interventions also varied from one time (deAraujo *et al*, 2010; Satoh *et al.*, 2009) to two times three months apart (Katzir *et al.*, 2010). Duration of the interventions ranged from minutes (deAraujo *et al*, 2010; Wells, 2010; Barax *et al.*, 2009) to one hour (Gardulf *et al.*, 2011). The interventionists across the studies varied greatly. A single nephrologist (Katzir *et al.*, 2010), dietitian (Morey *et al*, 2008; Kandiah *et al.*, 2010), social worker (Best *et al.*, 2010), nurse (Wells, 2011), or pharmacist (Satoh *et al.*, 2009) were used. Intervention teams consisted of nurses who care for both kidney and general patients (Baraz *et al.*,

2009; VanCamp *et al.*, 2011); dialysis nurses, technicians, dietitian, and social worker (Russell *et al.*, 2011); and a team of a registered nurse, dietitian, and nephrologist (Gardulf *et al.*, 2010). One study did not document the interventionist (de Aruajo *et al.*, 2010).

Medication and diet adherence outcomes were measured by phosphorus serum levels, self-report, or electronic monitoring. Serum levels were used alone in five studies (Kandiah *et al.*, 2010; Best *et al.*, 2011; Baraz *et al.*, 2009; de Araujo *et al.*, 2010; Satoh *et al.*, 2009). Self report alone was used in one study (Wells *et al.*, 2011). A combination of serum levels and self-report or self-report and electronic monitoring (Medication Electronic Monitoring System [MEMS], MEMS Track Cap, Apres Corp., Union City, CA, USA) were used in five studies (Morey *et al.*, 2008; Russell *et al.*, 2011; Van Camp *et al.*, 2011; Katzir *et al.*, 2010; Gardulf *et al.*, 2010). The KDOQI guidelines were used when assessing the serum phosphorus levels.

Of the eleven reviewed studies, seven studies (63.6%) had at least one statistically significant finding (Morey *et al.*, 2008; Katzir *et al.*, 2010; Gardulf *et al.*, 2011; Best *et al.*, 2011; Satoh *et al.*, 2009; Baraz *et al.*, 2009; Van Camp *et al.*, 2011). Of these seven statistically successful studies, four studies utilized a cognitive-behavioral approach (Morey *et al.*, 2008; Gardulf *et al.*, 2011; Best *et al.*, 2011; Van Camp *et al.*, 2011) while three studies employed a cognitive intervention (Katzir *et al.*, 2010; Satoh *et al.*, 2009; Baraz *et al.*, 2009).

The outcome focus of the seven successful studies was diet and medication adherence, fluid adherence and missed treatments (Tables **5** and **6**). Six studies improved adherence to diet and phosphate binding medication (Morey *et al.*, 2008; Katzir *et al.*, 2010; Gardulf *et al.*, 2011; Satoh *et al.*, 2009; Baraz *et al.*, 2009; and Van Camp *et al.*, 2011). In addition to diet adherence, Baraz *et al.*, (2009) also improved fluid adherence with their cognitive intervention. One successful study focused their cognitive-behavioral intervention towards improving missed treatments (Best *et al.*, 2011).

Table 5: Diet and Medication (Phosphorus) Adherence results.

Author	Intervention	Results
Baraz *et al.,* (2009)	Cognitive	**Phos +**
De Araujo *et al.,* (2010)	Cognitive	Phos – Calcium -
Katzir *et al.,* (2010)	Cognitive	**Self-report medication adherence +** Phosphorus – Calcium -
Sotah *et al.,* (2009)	Cognitive	Phos + **Ca/phos product +**
Gardulf *et al.,* (2010)	Cognitive-behavioral	Phos + Calcium – Albumin -
Kandiah *et al.,* (2010)	Cognitive-behavioral	Phos – Ca/phos product -
Morey *et al.,* (2008)	Cognitive-behavioral	Phos – Ca/phos - Self-report medication adherence -
Russell *et al.,* (2011)	Cognitive-behavioral	Phos – Albumin -
Van Camp *et al.,* (2011)	Cognitive-behavioral	**Phos +** **Calcium +** **Adherence+**
Wells (2011)	Cognitive-behavioral	Perceived medication adherence +

Abbreviations: Phos=Phosphorous; Ca/phos=calcium/phosphorous product; +=statistically significant; -=not statistically significant).

Table 6: Fluid and Dialysis Treatment (Kt/V or IDWG) Adherence results.

Author	Intervention	Results
Baraz *et al.,* (2009)	Cognitive	**IDWG +**
De Araujo *et al.,* (2010)	Cognitive	Kt/V -
Katzir *et al.,* (2010)	Cognitive	IDWG -
Best *et al.,* (2011)	Cognitive-behavioral	**Missed treatments +**
Russell *et al.,* (2011)	Cognitive-behavioral	Missed/shortened treatments – IDWG -

Abbreviations: IDWG= Inter-Dialytic Weight Gain; Kt/V= measure of dialysis adequacy; +=statistically significant; - =not statistically significant.

DISCUSSION

The purpose of this report is to systematically review the intervention studies from 2007-2012 which have attempted to enhance hemodialysis adherence in adults. Seven of the eleven studies (63.6%) had a statistically significant improvement in treatment, fluid, diet and/or medication adherence. In our 2008 review, six out of 8 studies (75%) had statistically significant results (Matteson & Russell, 2010). Though this review includes a small number of studies, the results surpass the findings from the general adherence intervention research in which statistically significant results were found in only about 50% of the studies (Haynes, *et al.*, 2005; Kripalani, Yao, & Haynes, 2007; McDonald, *et al.*, 2002; Roter, Hall, Merisca, Nordstrom, Cretin, & Svarstad, 1998). In this group of reviewed studies, cognitive interventions, involving primarily education, delivered in various formats, continues to be a prevalent adherence intervention with three of the five studies documenting statistically significant results. Prior studies have documented that education is necessary but not sufficient for adherence behavior change (Conn *et al.*, 2009).

Cognitive-behavioral interventions outnumbered cognitive interventions and had a greater number of successful studies enhancing adherence behaviors. The cognitive-behavioral interventions included motivation and self-care behaviors. Self-care behaviors have been shown to be a powerful intervention in medication adherence behavior change (Conn *et al.,* 2009). This finding is consistent with our initial review where cognitive-behavioral interventions were more successful (Matteson & Russell, 2010); however, in this review almost all of the studies used a quasi-experimental design, not the stronger randomized controlled trial design so comparisons are difficult.

The strength of the methodological reporting in this group of studies was varied. In evaluating the CONSORT data, the methods sections of the two RCT's were evaluated as the weakest area of reporting. The lowest STROBE score was Best *et al.,* (2011) which was an abstract, which limited the study details and consequently our ability to evelute the study details. Documenting study bias, study size determination, and missing data procedures were the main STROBE reporting deficiencies; however, result details were also lacking. Participant flow diagrams document participant drop out (stage of drop out and reason) and could have improved the STROBE scoring of the studies.

Interventions delivered by teams was a unique finding of this review. In our earlier review, most of the studies used solo interventionists (Matteson & Russell, 2010). Interventions are increasingly including teams of interventionists, possibly indicating a more inter-professional team approach to dialysis treatment adherence. An expert panel convened by the American Association of Colleges of Nursing and organizations representing medical, dental, pharmacy and public health recently published the "Core Competencies for Interprofessional Collaborative Practice Report". The purpose of this report is to provide intra-professional competences for students of these disciplines "so that they enter the workforce ready to practice effective teamwork and team-based care" (p. i) (Interprofessional Education Collaborative Expert Panel, 2011). Hemodiaysis interventions appear to be increasingly delivered using this intra-professional approach.

Strengths of the reviewed studies include the number of countries publishing research. The majority of the studies were published outside of the U.S., documenting that hemodialysis nonadherence is a world-wide problem and that researchers are responding to this complex problem by testing traditional cognitive and cognitive-behavioral interventions.

Many of the methodological weaknesses such as weak research designs, small sample sizes, brief interventions (dose and duration), few intervention details, inconsistent measurement instruments, and inconsistent measurement parameters continue to be present in the studies reviewed from 2007-2012. Only two RCTs have been published in the last five years. The number of published studies is encouraging, but researchers must use the randomized controlled trial design so that the evidence from the studies is of the highest quality (Polit, & Beck, 2012). Sample sizes of the majority of the reviewed studies were small and only three studies specifically targeted a nonadherent sample. Small, heterogenous samples can decrease the statistical power of a study by increasing the sampling error (Polit & Beck, 2012). Targeting the intervention to a nonadherent, homogenous sample allows smaller sample sizes with more potential for change; whereas, an adherent sample limits the difference due to the intervention, creating a 'ceiling' effect (Polit, & Beck, 2012).

The intervention dose and duration was brief with limited long-term follow-up. Increasing the dose and duration of the intervention with long-term follow-up may have a greater effect than an intervention administered one time. Intervention details were lacking and interventions could not be replicated based on the limited amount of information provided in the studies. Interventions should be described in detail so that studies can be replicated which adds to the body of knowledge through generalizability; according to Conn and Groves (2011). If interventions are poorly described, the progress of interventional research may be slowed by limiting the reproduction of the study (Conn, & Groves, 2011).

Inconsistent measurement of hemodialysis adherence continues to plague the hemodialysis adherence intervention literature. In the previous review, inconsistent adherence outcome measures were also utilized, which may not adequately reflect the patient's adherence to hemodialysis treatment, fluid, diet and medication adherence. For example, De Araujo (2010) used Kt/V as the fluid adherence outcome measure but Kt/V is also reflective of the nephrologist's skill in managing dialysis.

Self-report measures were used extensively in this group of reviewed studies compared to our previous review which threatens the validity of the results (Matteson, & Russell, 2010). The increase in the use of self-report measures over the last five years may be due to the ease of administration and the low cost of the measures; however, self-report often over-estimates adherence due to potential for mis-representation and social desirabilityreponse bias (Polit, & Beck, 2012). More valid measures of hemodialysis adherence outcomes are available. For example, medication adherence measurement could be standardized with the use of electronic monitoring; the MEMS cap has been utilized to measure medication adherence and has been found a valid and reliable measurement of medication adherence (Denhaerynck *et al.*, 2008; Riekert, 2002). Information technology has facilitated fluid/diet adherence self-monitoring and has been successful in both healthy and chronically ill patients and may assist in self-management of diet/fluid adherence behaviors possibly leading to improved hemodialysis outcomes (Welch *et al.*, 2010).

The differences five years have made are stark. The weakness of the studies included in Matteson and Russell (2010) review have continued. Studies still have weak research designs, small sample sizes, brief interventions (dose and duration), few intervention details, inconsistent measurement instruments, and inconsistent measurement parameters. Researchers must conduct fully-powered randomized controlled trial designs. Implementing fully powered studies are expensive and time consuming. Funding agencies are encouraged to offer grants that support these strong research designs.

Additionally, personal system-based interventions involving the system in which the patient functions has not been tested in this population, but has had large effect sizes in other chronic diseases (Russell, 2010; Matteson, & Russell, 2011). Through a data evaluation and system refinement process called Plan-Do-Check-Act, personal system changes are identified and implemented; health behaviors become ritualistic and habitual, with less effort, motivation, and intention required to maintain the desired health behavior change. This approach does not blame the individual for adherence problems but rather focuses on improving the personal system that creates and maintains the behavior (Alemi, & Neuhauser, 2006; Gustafson, Cats-Baril, & Alemi, 1992; Russell, 2010). "Interventions need to focus on both patient factors and the extent to which relationships and system problems compromise the patient's ability to adhere to medication and treatment plans" (p.479).(Kammerer, Garry, Hartigan, Carter, & Erlich, 2007). With cognitive and cognitive-behavioral interventions showing mixed results, we need to look towards an innovative intervention to enhance hemodialysis adherence.

CONCLUSIONS

In summary, eleven studies (two randomized controlled trial and nine quasi-experimental studies) were identified attempting to enhance hemodialysis adherence. This is a systematic review of intervention studies targeting treatment, diet, fluid, and medication adherence in adult hemodialysis patients from 2007 to 2012. Strengths and limitations of the studies are noted. Future studies should include a randomized controlled trial study design, a large, diverse nonadherent sample including multi-disciplinary teams as interventionists. Hemodialysis adherence interventions must be theory-based and address the system in which the patient functions to enhance adherence.

ACKNOWLEDGEMENT

None Declared.

CONFLICT OF INTEREST

None Declared.

REFERENCES

AARDEX Group, MEMS [apparatus and software]. 2011, Switzerland: Retrieved from http://www.aardexgroup.com/aardex_index.php?group=aardex&id=99.

Alemi, F., & Neuhauser, D. (Eds.). (2006). A thinking person's weight loss and exercise program. Fairfax, Virginia: George Mason University.

Baraz, S., Parvardeh, S., Mohammadi, E., & Broumand, B. (3009). Dietary and fluid compliance: An educational intervention for patients having haemodialysis. Journal of Advanced Nursing, 66(1), 60-68.

Best, S., Canny, B., Averette, E., Cameron, D., Keaveney, D,.Russ, H. (2011). Reducing behavior-based missed hemodialysis treatments. Nephrology Nursing Journal, 38(2), 194.

Block, G. A., Klassen, P. S., Lazarus, J. M., Ofsthun, N., Lowrie, E. G., & Chertow, G. M. (2004). Mineral metabolism, mortality, and morbidity in maintenance hemodialysis. J Am Soc Nephrol, 15(8), 2208-2218. doi: 10.1097/01.ASN.0000133041.27682.A2.

Conn, V. S., Hafdahl, A. R., Cooper, P. S., Ruppar, T. M., Mehr, D. R., & Russell, C. L. (2009). Interventions to improve medication adherence among older adults: meta-analysis of adherence outcomes among randomized controlled trials. Gerontologist, 49(4), 447-462. doi: gnp037 [pii] 10.1093/geront/gnp037.

Conn, V. S., & Groves, P. S. (2011). Protecting the power of interventions through proper reporting. [Review]. Nurs Outlook, 59(6), 318-325. doi: 10.1016/j.outlook.2011.06.003.

de Araujo, L., Figueiredo, A. & d'Avila, D. (2010). Evaluation of an educational program on calcium and phosphorus metabolism for patients on hemodialysis. Rev Esc Enferm USP, 44(4), 927-931.

Denhaerynck, K., Schafer-Keller, P., Young, J., Steiger, J., Bock, A., & De Geest, S. (2008). Examining assumptions regarding valid electronic monitoring of medication therapy: development of a validation framework and its application on a European sample of kidney transplant patients. BMC Med Res Methodol, 8, 5. doi: 1471-2288-8-5 [pii] 10.1186/1471-2288-8-5.

Gardulf, A., Palsson, M., & Nicolay, U. (2011). Education for dialysis patients lowers long-term phosphate levels and maintains healthrelated quality of life. Clinical Nephrology, 75(4), 319-327.

Gustafson, D. H., Cats-Baril, W. L., & Alemi, F. (1992). Systems to support health policy analysis: theory, models, and uses. Ann Arbor, Mich.: Health Administration Press.

Interprofessional Education Collaborative Expert Panel. (2011). Core competencies for interprofessional collaborative practice: Report of an expert panel. Washington, D.C.: Interprofessional Education Collaborative.

Kammerer, J., Garry, G., Hartigan, M., Carter, B., & Erlich, L. (2007). Adherence in patients on dialysis: strategies for success. [Review]. Nephrol Nurs J, 34(5), 479-486.

Kandiah, J., Resler, J., & Amend, V. (2010). Effects of an innovative educational contest to lower serum phosphorous levels and calcium-phosphorous products in hemodialysis patients. Topics in Clinical Nutrition, 25(4), 345-350.

Karamanidou, C., Clatworthy, J., Weinman, J., & Horne, R. (2008). A systematic review of the prevalence and determinants of nonadherence to phosphate binding medication in patients with end-stage renal disease. [Comparative Study Research Support, Non-U.S. Gov't Review]. BMC Nephrol, 9, 2. doi: 10.1186/1471-2369-9-2.

Katzir, Z., Boaz, M., Backshi, I., Cernes, R., Barnea, Z., & Biro, A. (2010). Medication apprehension and compliance among dialysis patients--a comprehensive guidance attitude. Nephron Clin Pract, 114(2), c151-157. doi: 10.1159/000254388.

Kim, Y., & Evangelista, L. S. (2010). Relationship between illness perceptions, treatment adherence, and clinical outcomes in patients on maintenance hemodialysis. Nephrol Nurs J, 37(3), 271-280; quiz 281.

Kripalani, S., Yao, X., Haynes, R. B. (2007). Interventions to Enhance Medication Adherence in Chronic Medical Conditions: A Systematic Review. Archives of Internal Medicine, 167(6), 540-550.

Kugler, C., Maeding, I., & Russell, C. L. (2011). Non-adherence in patients on chronic hemodialysis: an international comparison study. [Comparative Study Multicenter Study Research Support, Non-U.S. Gov't]. J Nephrol, 24(3), 366-375. doi: 10.5301/JN.2010.5823.

Leggat, J. E., Jr., Orzol, S. M., Hulbert-Shearon, T. E., Golper, T. A., Jones, C. A., Held, P. J., & Port, F. K. (1998). Noncompliance in hemodialysis: predictors and survival analysis. Am J Kidney Dis, 32(1), 139-145.

Matteson, M. L., & Russell, C. (2010). Interventions to improve hemodialysis adherence: a systematic review of randomized-controlled trials. [Review]. Hemodial Int, 14(4), 370-382. doi: 10.1111/j.1542-4758.2010.00462.x

McDonald, H. P. B., Garg, A. X. M. D. M. A., & Haynes, R. B. M. D. P. (2002). Interventions to Enhance Patient Adherence to Medication Prescriptions: Scientific Review. JAMA, 288(22), 2868-2879.

Morey, B., Walker, R., & Davenport, A. (2008). More dietetic time, Better outcome? A randomized prospective study investigating the effect of more dietetic time on phosphate control in end-stage kidney failure haemodialysis patients. Nephron Clinical Practice, 109, c173-180.

Obialo, C. I., Hunt, W.C., Bashir, W., & Zager, P.G. (2012). Relationship of missed and shortened hemodialysis treatments to hospitalization and mortality: observations from a US dialysis network. Clinical Kidney Journal, 5, 315-319.

Peterson, A. M., Takiya, L., & Finley, R. (2003). Meta-analysis of trials of interventions to improve medication adherence. Am J Health Syst Pharm, 60(7), 657-665.

Polit, D. F., Beck, C.T. (2012). Nursing Research: Generating and assessing evidence for nursing practice (9th ed.). Philadelphia, PA: Wolters Kluwer/Lippincott Williams & Wilkins.

Riekert, K. A. R., C.S. (2002). Electronic monitoring of medication adherence: When is high-tech best? Journal of Clinical Psychology in Medical Settings, 9(1), 25-34.

Roter, D. L., Hall, J., Merisca, R., Nordstrom, B., Cretin, D., & Svarstad, B. (1998). Effectiveness of Interventions to Improve Patient Compliance: A Meta-Analysis. Medical Care, 36(8), 1138-1161.

Russell, C. L., Whitlock, R., Knowles, N., Peace, L., Tanner, B., Hong, B. A. (2008). Rates and correlates of therapy non-adherence in adult hemodialysis patients. Journal of Nephrology Social Work, 28, 11-17.

Russell, C. L. (2010). A clinical nurse specialist-led intervention to enhance medication adherence using the plan-do-check-act cycle for continuous self-improvement. Clin Nurse Spec, 24(2), 69-75. doi: 10.1097/NUR.0b013e3181cf554d.

Russell, C. L., Cronk, N. J., Herron, M., Knowles, N., Matteson, M. L., Peace, L., & Ponferrada, L. (2011). Motivational Interviewing in Dialysis Adherence Study (MIDAS). [Research Support, Non-U.S. Gov't]. Nephrol Nurs J, 38(3), 229-236.

Sabaté, E. & World Health Organization (2003). Adherence to long-term therapies : evidence for action. Geneva: World Health Organization.

Saran, R., Bragg-Gresham, J. L., Rayner, H. C., Goodkin, D. A., Keen, M. L., Van Dijk, P. C., Port, F. K. (2003). Nonadherence in hemodialysis: associations with mortality, hospitalization, and practice patterns in the DOPPS. Kidney Int, 64(1), 254-262. doi: 10.1046/j.1523-1755.2003.00064.x.

Satoh, M., Koizumi, A., Izumi, S., Kugoh, Y., Kiriyama, E.,.Hirata, S. (2009). Improvement of hyperphosphatemia following patient education. Journal of Pharm Technology, 25, 3-9.

Schulz, K. F., Altman, D. G., & Moher, D. (2010). CONSORT 2010 statement: updated guidelines for reporting parallel group randomized trials. Obstet Gynecol, 115(5), 1063-1070. doi: 10.1097/AOG.0b013e3181d9d421 00006250-201005000-00028 [pii].

U S Renal Data System, USRDS 2012 Annual Data Report: Atlas of Chronic Kidney Disease and End-Stage Renal Disease in the United States, National Institutes of Health, National Institute of Diabetes and Digestive and Kidney Diseases, Bethesda, MD, 2012.

Van Camp, Y., Huybrechts, S. A., Van Rompaey, B., & Elseviers, M. M. (2011). Nurse-led education and counselling to enhance adherence to phospate binders. Journal of Clinical Nursing, 21, 1304-1313.

von Elm, E., Altman, D. G., Egger, M., Pocock, S. J., Gotzsche, P. C., & Vandenbroucke, J. P. (2007). The Strengthening the Reporting of Observational Studies in Epidemiology (STROBE) statement: guidelines for reporting observational studies. Lancet, 370(9596), 1453-1457. doi: S0140-6736(07)61602-X [pii] 10.1016/S0140-6736(07)61602-X.

Welch, J. L., Siek, K.A., Connelly, K.H., Astroth, K.S., McManus, M.S., Scott, L., Heo, S., Kraus, M.A. (2010). Merging health literacy with computer technology: Self-management diet and fluid intake among adult hemodialysis patients. Patient Education and Counseling, 79, 192-198.

Wells, J. R. (2011). Hemodialysis knowledge and medical adherence in African Americans diagnosed with end stage renal disease: results of an educational intervention. [Research Support, Non-U.S. Gov't Review]. Nephrol Nurs J, 38(2), 155-162; quiz 163.

Send Orders of Reprints at reprints@benthamscience.net

CHAPTER 9

Evaluating the Psychological Burden and Quality of Life in Caregivers of Patients Under Dialysis

Georgios K. Tzitzikos[1,*] and Constantinos M. Togas[2]

[1]*General Hospital of Corinth, Renal Department, Hellas, Greece and* [2]*Ministry of Justice, Hellas, Greece*

Abstract: Patients with end-stage kideny disease (ESKD) and their caregivers follow a rigorous program for the needs of treatment with daily restrictions and significant impact on their lifestyle. In this process, psychosocial factors (educational level, economic status, family, supportive environment) are involved, that interact with each other, influencing the subjective experience of disease, while they hinder or facilitate the adjustment of the individual to the new conditions. Caregivers are usually family members who agree to give systematic priority to the patient's needs, neglecting their own, thus becoming vulnerable. Caregivers carry an increased psychological burden, and are often prone to stress, anxiety and depression, and their health appears to be compromised. Studies conducted so far show that caregivers of dialysis patients experience isolation have diminished confidence and express exhaustion, and generally have low quality of life. Nevertheless, there are mixed results regarding the extent and severity of impact on their lives and health. Researchers seem to agree that the most important factor affecting caregivers is the patient's health status. The role of caregivers is often invisible and not recognized. To enable caregivers to cope with the burden borne, support services in the form of consultancy, training, social care or home care, where appropriate, should be obtained.

Keywords: Caregivers, carers, family, end-stage kidney disease, kidney disease, eskd, burden, needs, experience, dialysis, dialysis caregivers, dialysis patients,caregivers' burden, caregivers' qol, caregivers' depression, caregivers' health, family caregivers, informal caregivers, caregivers' mental health, chronic renal failure, caregivers of children with renal failure, caregivers' psychopathology, caregivers' stress, renal replacement therapy.

INTRODUCTION

The Greek philosopher Antisthenes has expressed the view that "the investigation of the meaning of words is the beginning of education".

*Address correspondence to Georgios Tzitzikos:** General Hospital of Corinth, Renal Department, Hellas, Greece; Tel: +0030 2741361832; Fax: +0030 2741020529; E-mail: tzitzikos1@gmail.com

Finding the meaning of the word 'care', we see that in different cultures it is listed as a multidimensional mental and emotional state, in which as a verb, it can mean among other things- "feel concern or interest", "attach importance to something", or "look after" and "provide for the needs of". As a noun: "the provision of what is necessary for the health, welfare, maintenance, and protection of someone or something" (Oxford dictionaries, 2012). These concepts often coexist, supporting Van Manen's (2000) notice, that "the more I care for this other, the more I worry and the stronger my desire to care". In human history, 'caring' has always been a fundamental component of the cohesion of the family and, by extension, of society, and it was always linked with feelings of love, solidarity and sense of duty.

Caring is an expression of respect and responds to human values as well as helps both the person who receives it and the person who offers it (Mayeroff, 1971). So, for some people, the meaning of care may be that of life itself.

The main recipients of care are always children, the elderly and patients or disabled persons of all ages, namely those unable to cope independently with everyday needs. Especially patients, under the influence of uncertainty about the outcome of the disease, have often more needs that extend beyond their psychology level, to the social dimension of life (Kimmel, 2000).

Caregivers can be identified as the persons most closely involved in patients' care, who try to help them to cope with the demands and circumstances of the disease. They are also known as informal or family caregivers, because they are not professionals, but members of the close family, especially first-degree relatives. Caregivers devote time every day, spending an average of 20 hours per week offering substantial assistance to cover patient's basic daily needs (National Alliance for Caregiving, 2009). In fact, they also offer emotional support to the patient, by giving him/her the strength to face the daily adversities of the disease. Furthermore, caregivers are often the missing link that connects patients with the outside world, helping them with basic daily activities such as communication with family and friends, orientation within the healthcare system, management of financial affairs, supplies of goods and home maintenance. In summary, the caregiver becomes the patient's arm that supports all aspects of life during the disease.

In the modern world, although the increasing demand for larger, more complex and specialized health services often leads in professionals taking the role of caregiver, family caregivers continue to cover the wider range of needs, to the patients' benefit. It is estimated that in the U.S. alone, 29% of the population, that is more than 65 million people, provide care for a chronically ill, disabled or aged family member or friend, and their services contribute to saving the health systems huge amounts of money. At the same time, families are forced to shoulder significant costs, which are required by the patient's condition, resulting in significant restriction of their economic potential. It is characteristic that a family spends on a child with special health problems on average three times more money, compared to a family with a healthy child (Newacheck, & Kim, 2005).

Oftentimes, the need for care can easily exceed the physical and mental limits of the caregiver, leading to a chronic stressful situation, known as the "caregiver burden" (Zarit, 2002), which makes caregivers suffer.

The burden can be objective when it refers to factors such as time spent on care, the economic costs or the tasks the caregiver has to carry out, and subjective when it comes to how the caregiver perceives the impact of the objective burden (Montgomery *et al.*, 1985).

Surveys show that caregivers may have impaired physical and mental health, and persons who were experiencing caregiver strain had a 63% higher mortality risk compared with a control group who were not caregivers (Schulz, & Beach, 1999). Caregivers, because of the burden, may have problems for which they may require health services for themselves, thus increasing the overall care needs, which the health system should offer. It is understood that the direct and indirect effects of caregiver burden are negative for all involved, and more broadly consist of chronic social, political and health problems that could be prevented or eliminated by applying an appropriate strategy (Garces *et al.*, 2003).

One of the most serious chronic diseases is end-stage kidney disease (ESKD). Patients suffering from ESKD have to cope with many adversities, *e.g.,* physical symptoms, limitations in food and fluid intake, changes in their body image, work and economic status, social roles, activity levels, self - image, health status and normal routines, while their control over treatment cannot always be predicted (Theofilou, 2011; Theofilou, 2012; Theofilou, 2012a). Such constraints are expected to affect the patients' life and physical as well as social functioning, leading them to reconsider their personal and professional goals within the context of living with a chronic illness (Theofilou, 2012b; Theofilou, Synodinou, & Panagiotaki, 2013; Theofilou, 2012c).

In order to survive, ESKD patients undergo replacement therapies of renal function, which are complex and demanding. Compared with the past, the circumstances of replacement therapy of renal function have matured and there is a clear progress in many fields, so several objective factors that may affect caregivers have been improved (USRDS, 2011).

The treatment is safer, thanks to improved and more user friendly technologies used in dialysis. Also, the efficiency of treatment is increased by improved dialysis filters and the use of drugs that allow patient to maintain his/her condition more stable. The observed reduction in mortality rates of patients creates the need for more long-term care, and a parallel reduction in hospitalization days shifts the focus of care on home and family caregivers (USRDS, 2011).

The difficulties encountered in providing appropriate care to patients with chronic renal failure, have been claimed to be proportional to the difficulties of any chronic disease and can cause a significant burden on persons who are directly responsible for providing care, particularly when they are family members (Cantor 1983; Belasco *et al.*, 2006). But in reality, chronic renal failure differs substantially from other chronic diseases, especially according to the mode chosen to replace renal function. In renal replacement therapy at home, either hemodialysis or peritoneal dialysis, patients and caregivers shoulder bigger responsibilities. The implementation of treatment requires special knowledge and skills as well as the ability to manage many different medicinal products, creating a situation that could result in caregivers' stress, anxiety, fatigue and emotional disorders. Family relationships are also likely to worsen and limit social contacts of family members (Beanlands *et al.*, 2005).

Renal replacement therapy in a dialysis center can provide a greater sense of safety, both to patients and caregivers, since the responsibility of dialysis and the monitoring of patient is undertaken by health professionals. However, the patient has to move to and from the dialysis unit frequently for therapy, which requires adherence to a strict time frame, something that drastically reduces other family activities and may result in interfamilial tensions and frictions (Rau-Foster, 2001; Molumphy, & Sporakowski, 1984).

Therefore, this chapter will draw on the key literature in this field as identified by psychiatric, medical and social sciences databases, with the aim to conduct a systematic review which explores the psychological burden and quality of life in ESKD patients' caregivers.

METHOD

In order to approach the psychological burden and quality of life in caregivers of patients with ESKD, we searched the literature during the last 30 years (from 1983 to 2012) in electronic databases such as pubmed/medline, sciencedirect, PyscINFO, google scholar, and scirus, for related publications in journals and books, but also relative sites, including the following terms: caregivers; carers; family; end-stage renal/kidney disease; ESKD; burden; needs; experience; dialysis. After reading the titles of references that appeared, we made a primary index of 674 articles, of which 49 or 36 were finally selected on the topic. Table **1** summarizes the studies included in the review

All the available reviews and research studies related to caregivers of the dialysis patients till 2012 were included. In the relevant studies found to date, quantitative studies have been conducted by using a wide variety of instruments, in order to measure the burden, the depression, and the quality of life of caregivers of dialysis patients; From the quantitative studies, it was found that most of them were cross-sectional (16), although there were two longitudinal ones, and in three studies a control group was used.

Five qualitative studies on caregivers of dialysis patients were also found, which will be discussed below, while there are six reviews of previous similar studies.

MAIN FINDINGS

Caregivers themselves, in an informal but interesting report in American Association of Kidney Patients (AAKP), argue that they have not enough time for their own activities and that they need space to relax. Also, they feel helpless when they are "unable to make the situation better or the pain go away" and "overwhelmed with responsibility" or "unable to share feelings and concerns with others". Furthermore, handling the daily financial responsibilities and arrangements is stressful (American Association of Kidney Patients, 2012).

Measuring quality of life of caregivers of elderly patients undergoing hemodialysis or peritoneal dialysis, it was observed that 1/3 of them indicated signs of depression, as well as a significant burden with negative impact on their quality of life, especially those who care for patients under peritoneal dialysis (Belasco *et al.*, 2006).

In a multicenter survey in Spain, quality of life of caregivers (Alvarez *et al.*, 2004) seems to be slightly worse compared to the general population. The authors also noted that younger caregivers are those who experience a greater burden, poorer quality of life and increased risk of depression.

Further, a study involving 50 elderly patients receiving dialysis (Parlevliet *et al.*, 2012), indicated that 84.4% of caregivers feel a heavy burden because of their patients' condition.

Additionally, in a survey conducted in Chile which involved 162 patients and their caregivers, it was found that a large percentage of them (over 40% in both groups) had symptoms of depression (Arechabala *et al.*, 2011).

The burden experienced by caregivers of patients on peritoneal dialysis in Japan, appears to be lower than the burden of caregivers of patients with dementia or stroke. However, quality of life compared to the general population, shows markedly lower assessments in indicators such as mental health and sociability (Shimoyama *et al.*, 2003).

Rioux *et al.,* (2012) in a study including 61 patients treated with nocturnal peritoneal dialysis and their caregivers, found that for both groups there were significant signs of depression, although the total burden is low, both for patients and caregivers.

According to Suri *et al.*, (2011), patients who are practicing in Frequent Hemodialysis Network (FHN), are believed to cause a significant burden on their family caregivers, while they themselves experience another burden related to depression and worse quality of life. Significant burden on caregivers and negative impact on their quality of life is also shown by a similar study in 100 caregivers of dialysis patients in Brazil (Belasco, 2002). Nevertheless, other studies with regards to African-American caregivers of dialysis patients showed that the majority of them assess their health as good. Also, 65% of participants had no signs of clinical depression, 14.7% showed mild distress, 14.7% indicated moderate distress, and only 4.0% had scores that corresponded to severe distress (Byers *et al.*, 2011).

In another study conducted in Turkey in 130 caregivers of patients under peritoneal dialysis, no experiences of loneliness and depression were observed (Asti *et al.*, 2006). Similarly, in a study by Wicks *et al.*, (1997), regarding 96 caregivers of ESKD patients, good quality of life was reported, which correlates to the absence of burden. The researchers also note that the burden and the caregivers' quality of life did not differ according to race and gender of the caregiver or patient, or the caregiver's relation to the patient, or even according to the type of renal replacement therapy.

A study which gives similar results (Harris *et al.*, 2000) in 78 young African-American caregivers showed that 68% of them feel to have little or no burden at all.

A survey to investigate the depression of caregivers of elderly hemodialysis patients, (Matsuu *et al.*, 2001) argues that caregivers may feel heavy burden because they are forced to cope with a special role in patient's life, but the authors also note that there is no difference in the occurrence of depression compared to controls who participated in the survey.

In a cross-sectional survey, not yet published, the psychological features of 106 caregivers of hemodialysis patients in Greece were investigated, regarding the experiences of shame, hostility, anxiety and symptoms of psychopathology. Compared to the general population, caregivers surveyed did not show higher scores on the respective scales, except the hostility one. In some cases, a mild psychological burden in caregivers was recorded, but it seems to be correlated to age and educational level and not to the nature of their duties (Tzitzikos, 2010).

By examining 50 hemodialysis patients and caregivers for emotional stability and manifestations of anxiety and depression, Ferrario *et al.,* (2002) found that patients suffer from significant stress, while caregivers showed a good emotional stability and low burden.

In an interesting cohort study using questionnaires about quality of life, it was found that at the beginning of dialysis both patients and their caregivers had impaired quality of life and there was a significant correlation to co-morbidity and functional ability of the patient. But after one year, the quality of life scores showed improvement, especially in the domain of social functioning (Fan *et al.,* 2008).

The functional impairment of the patient as a factor negatively affecting caregivers is highlighted in a study of 38 home hemodialysis patients and their caregivers (Piira *et al.,* 2002). Here, the authors by examining the cognitive factors, they observed that caregivers who had external locus of control and were more focused on emotion, reported a higher negative effect.

An evaluation of mental health involving 30 caregivers of hemodialysis patients in Poland (Klak *et al.,* 2008) indicated that 87% of the participants had signs of mental disorder (derangement) and increased burden, which is correlated to exhaustion, negative emotions and lack of energy. In addition, it was found that the burden was higher for caregivers of more demented patients. Even a recent study that assessed 142 patients and caregivers, suggests that caregivers of hemodialysis patients experience an adverse quality of life. In the same study the caregivers appear to have also poor sleep quality (Çelik *et al.,* 2012).

Blogg, & Hyde (2008) in a qualitative study using an ethnological approach of caregivers in home hemodialysis patients, report that the burden of care may vary from person to person, and the most aggravating of all factors for the caregiver is the health status of the patient.

Two separate qualitative studies have employed the phenomenological approach. Luk (2002) argues that caring for home dialysis patients in China, entails economic, emotional, social and health-related impacts. Regarding the bio-psycho-social impact of ESKD and experiences that causes, while White, & Grenyer (1999) noted that although both patients and their partners have a positive view of their relationship, they both are overwhelmed by the impact of hemodialysis on their lives.

Another study (Pelletier-Hibbert, & Sohi 2001) gleans experiences of family members of hemodialysis patients through interviews, approaching the factors of uncertainty, which are entering family life and cause stress. It appears that the good health condition of the patient and the existence of positive perspectives, such as a transplant, can play a positive role. Family members of patients avoid long-term plans and the whole situation seems to be more tolerable, when they address life with hope and faith.

Ziegert *et al.,* (2006) by interviewing thirteen caregivers, found that uninterrupted/continuous care to patients pushes caregivers to neglect their own health and become vulnerable. In contrast, those who are able to rest and take care of themselves, seem to be better shielded against health problems. In an attempt to measure the psychosocial needs of families of dialysis patients in a very small sample of participants (n= 10), the need for information and comfort emerged as a very important factor (Wagner, 1996).

Caregivers of Children with ESKD

Children are always the most sensitive part of the society and thus the care for their health is a high priority, especially for parents. There are not many children with chronic renal disease, but they have several health problems that make them vulnerable and directly affect their families.

Watson (1997) conducted a longitudinal study in two centers (U.S., UK) where he studied over time 24 families of children with chronic renal failure (CRF) regarding stress, anxiety and depression with the use of relevant questionnaires. Compared to fathers it appears that mothers are more impaired as their stress levels are above the normal and many of them are at borderline anxiety disorder level. Also, parents of older children seem to have more stress than those of younger children.

Similar results were found in a cross-sectional study (Wiedebusch *et al.*, 2010) including 195 parents of children with renal failure. It was found that mothers experience lower quality of life and higher psychosocial burden than fathers. Examining quality of life in children with renal failure and also their parents', McKenna *et al.,* (2006) found that parents have worse indicators than children in all domains. Children rated their quality of life lower than healthy controls, but higher than expected.

In a case-control study involving caregivers of 32 children under peritoneal dialysis in Taiwan, (Tsai *et al.*, 2003), it was found that the probability of depression was significantly higher in comparison to other groups of children. The mean scores for the quality of life in the study group were significantly lower in the domains of physical, psychological, social relationship, and environment quality.

Signs of depression, anxiety and high stress levels were observed in a review of 11 articles (Aldridge, 2008), about families who have children with renal failure. The author indicates that parents with lower socioeconomic status have more difficulty to settle the obligations arising from the illness of their children.

In a qualitative study of 20 parents conducted by Tong *et al.,* (2010), the authors aptly highlight the double parental role as a parent and as a provider of health services as well, and identify four main stages of caring for children: absorbing the clinical environment, meeting the role of caregiver, disruption of family routine/norms and finally coping with strategies and support structures.

The same authors also highlight the demanding role of parents raising children with chronic renal failure where 3 sections are identified/differentiated: the intrapersonal which refers to living with factors such as stress and uncertainty, the interpersonal where the role of parent is enlarged by incorporating the role of health provider, and the "external issues" relating to the management of liabilities incurred (Tong *et al.*, 2010).

Table 1: Overview of selected studies regarding psychological burden and quality of life in caregivers of patients under dialysis.

Author	Title	Journal	Type of study-Methodology	Patients/caregivers	Research tools
Aldridge, M.D. (2008).	How do families adjust to having a child with chronic kidney failure?	Nephrol Nurs J, 35(2): 157-62.	systematic review	Not stated	Not stated
Alvarez-Ude F *et al.* (2004)	Health-related quality of life of family caregivers of dialysis patients.	J Nephrol., 17(6): 841-50.	Cross-sectional	221 patients/. 221 caregiver	Short-Form Health Survey (SF-36), Duke-UNC Functional Social Support Questionnaire (FSS), Zarit Burden Interview (ZBI)
Arechabala *et al.,* (2011)	Depression and self-perceived burden of care by hemodialysis patients and their caregivers.	Rev Panam Salud Publica, 30(1): 74-79.	Descriptive and correlational	162 patients and their caregivers	Multidimensional Scale of Perceived Social Support; Self-perceived Burden Scale; Center for Epidemiologic Studies Depression Scale; Fatigue Severity Scale
Asti T *et al.,* (2006)	The experiences of loneliness, depression, and social support of Turkish patients with continuous ambulatory peritoneal dialysis and their caregivers.	J Clin Nurs. 15(4): 490-7.	Cross-sectional (Descriptive correlational design)	65 patients/. 65 caregivers	UCLA loneliness scale, Beck's depression scale, The perceived social support from family and friends scales.
Beanlands *et al.,* (2005)	Caregiving by family and friends of adults receiving dialysis.	Nephrol Nurs J; 32: 621–631.	Qualitative/ Interviews	37 caregivers	Not stated
Belasco A *et al.,* (2006)	Quality of life of family caregivers of elderly patients on hemodialysis and peritoneal dialysis.	Am J Kidney Dis., 48(6): 955-63.	Cross-sectional	124 caregivers/. 77 caregivers	Short-Form Health Survey (SF-36), Caregiver Burden scale, Cognitive Index of Depression.

Table 1: contd....

Belasco AG & Sesso R.(2002)	Burden and quality of life of caregivers for hemodialysis patients	American Journal of Kidney Diseases, 39 (4): 805-812.	Cross-sectional	100 patients/ 100 caregivers	Short-Form Health Survey (SF-36), Caregiver Burden scale
Blogg & Hyde (2008)	The experience of spouses caring for a person on home haemodialysis: an ethnography	Ren Soc Aust J, 4(3) 75-80.	Ethnographic methodology	5 caregivers	Not stated
Byers DJ *et al.,* (2011)	Depressive symptoms and health promotion behaviors of African-American women who are family caregivers of hemodialysis recipients.	Nephrol Nurs J, 38(5): 425-30.	Cross-sectional	75 caregivers	Center for Epidemiological Studies Depression Scale (CES-D), Severity of Caregiver's Disease Scale.
Celik G. *et al.,* (2012)	Are sleep and life quality of family caregivers affected as much as those of hemodialysis patients?	General Hospital Psychiatry, 34 (5): 518–524.	Cross-sectional	142 patients/. 142 caregivers	Short-Form Health Survey (SF-36). Pittsburgh Sleep Quality Index (PSQI), Hospital Anxiety and Depression Scale
Cukor D. *et al.,* (2007)	Psychosocial Aspects of Chronic Disease: ESRD as a Paradigmatic Illness	JASN, 18(12): 3042-3055	Review	Not stated	Not stated
Fan SL *et al.,* (2008)	Quality of life of caregivers and patients on peritoneal dialysis	Nephrology Dialysis Transplantation, 23 (5): 1713-1719.	Cohort Study	Not stated	Short-Form Health Survey (SF-36)
Ferrario SR *et al.,* (2002)	Emotional reactions and practical problems of the caregivers of hemodialysed patients.	J Nephrol., 5(1): 54-60.	Cross-sectional	50 patients/. 50 caregivers	Not stated
Gayomali Ch. *et al.,* (2008)	The challenge for the caregiver of the patient with chronic kidney disease	Nephrology Dialysis Transplantation, 23, (12): 3749-3751.	Review	Not stated	Not stated
Harris TT. *et al.,* (2000)	Subjective burden in young and older African-American caregivers of patients with end stage renal disease awaiting transplant.	Nephrol Nurs J., 27(4): 383-91; 355; discussion 392, 405.	Longitudinal	78 caregivers	22-item self-administered Burden Interview (BI)

Table 1: contd….

Klak R. *et al.*, (2008)	Exhaustion of caregivers of patients on maintenance haemodialysis.	Nephrology Dialysis Transplantation, 23(12): 4086.	Cross-sectional	30 caregivers	General Health Questionnaire (GHQ-12), Questionnaire of Caregiver's Burden (QCB), Mini-Mental State Examination (MMSE).
Low J. *et al.*, (2008)	The impact of end-stage kidney disease (ESKD) on close persons: a literature review.	Clinical Kidney Journal, 1(2): 67-79.	Literature review	Not stated	Not stated
Luk WS (2002)	The home care experience as perceived by the caregivers of Chinese dialysis patients	International Journal of Nursing Studies, 39(3): 269–277.	Qualitative/ Interviews	30 caregivers	Not stated
Matsuu *et al.*, (2001)	Depression among caregivers of elderly patients on chronic hemodialysis.	Fukuoka Igaku Zasshi; 2001; 92(9): 319-25.	Cross-sectional	Not stated	Center for Epidemiologic Studies Depression Scale evaluation (CESD)
McKenna Am. *et al.*, (2006)	Quality of life in children with chronic kidney dise ase-patient and caregiver assessments.	Nephrology Dialysis Transplantation, 21(7): 1899-1905.	Cross-sectional	59 patients (children)/. 58 caregivers	PedsQL Generic Core Scale
Parlevliet JL *et al.*, (2012)	Systematic comprehensive geriatric assessment in elderly patients on chronic dialysis: a cross-sectional comparative and feasibility study.	BMC Nephrology, 2012; 13: 30.	Cross-sectional	50 patients	Comprehensive Geriatric Assessment (CGA)
Pelletier-Hibbert M. & Sohi P. (2001)	Sources of uncertainty and coping strategies used by family members of individuals living with end stage renal disease.	Nephrology Nursing Journal, 28(4): 411-419.	Qualitative/ Interviews	41 caregivers	Not stated
Piira T. *et al.*, (2002)	The role of cognitive factors in the adjustment of home dialysis carers.	Psychology & Health, 17: 313-322.	Cross-sectional	38 patients/. 38 caregivers	Not stated

Table 1: contd....

Rioux *et al.,* (2012)	Caregiver burden among nocturnal home hemodialysis patients.	Hemodial Int, 16(2): 214-9.	Cross-sectional	36 patients/. 31 caregivers	Short Form Health Survey (SF-12), Beck Depression Inventory, Caregiver Burden scale
Shimoyama S *et al.,* (2003)	Health-related quality of life and caregiver burden among peritoneal dialysis patients and their family caregivers in Japan.	Perit Dial Int, 23(2): 200-205.	Cross-sectional	26 patients/. 34 caregivers	Kidney Disease Quality of Life Short Form (KDQOL-SF), Short-Form Health Survey (SF-36), Zarit Burden Interview (ZBI)
Suri *et al.,* (2011)	Burden on caregivers as perceived by hemodialysis patients in the Frequent Hemodialysis Network (FHN) trials	Nephrol. Dial. Transplant; 26(7): 2316-2322.	cross-sectional	412 participants	Cousineau Perceived Burden Scale
Tzitzikos G. (2010)	Psychological features of caregivers of dialysis patients	Master's thesis. University of Thessaly, Greece.	Cross-sectional	106 caregivers	Other As Shamer Scale (OAS); Hostility-Direction of Hostility Questionnaire (HDHQ); State - Trait Anxiety Inventory (STAI); Experience of Shame Scale (ESS); Symptom Check List -90 (SCL -90).
Tong A. *et al.,* (2008).	Experiences of Parents Who Have Children With Chronic Kidney Disease: A Systematic Review of Qualitative Studies	Pediatrics, 121(2): 349 -360.	Systematic review	Not stated	Not stated
Tong A. *et al.,* (2008)	Support interventions for caregivers of people with chronic kidney disease: a systematic review	Nephrology Dialysis Transplantation, 23, (12): 3960-3965.	Review	Not stated	Not stated

Table 1: contd….

Tong A *et al.,* (2010)	Parental perspectives on caring for a child with chronic kidney dise ase: an in-depth interview study	Child: Care, Health and Development, 36(4): 549–557.	Qualitative/ Interviews	20 patients	Not stated
Tsai TC. *et al.,* (2006)	Psychosocial effects on caregivers for children on chronic peritoneal dialysis	Kidney International, 70, 1983–1987.	Case-control	32 caregivers	The Taiwanese Depression Questionnaire, The World Health Organization QOL BRIEF-Taiwan Version.
Wagner CD. (1996)	Family needs of chronic hemodialysis patients: a comparison of perceptions of nurses and families.	ANNA J., 23(1): 19-26; 27-8.	Qualitative/ Interviews	10 family members /. 9 nurses	The Norris and Grove Questionnaire (1986) (modified for the hemodialysis population)
Watson AR (1997)	Stress and Burden of Care in Families with Children Commencing Renal Replacement Therapy	Adv Perit Dial., 13: 300-4.	Longitudinal	38 patients	Not stated
White Y & Grenyer BF(1999)	The biopsychosocial impact of end-stage renal disease: the experience of dialysis patients and their partner	Journal of Advanced Nursing, 30(6): 1312–1320.	Qualitative/ Interviews	22 caregivers/ . 22 patients	Not stated
Wicks MN *et al.,* (1997)	Subjective burden and quality of life in family caregivers of patients with end stage renal disease.	ANNA J., 24(5): 527-8; 531-8; 539-40.	Exploratory descriptive desig n	96 patients/. 96 caregivers	Caregiver Burden Interview, General QoL measure.
Wiedebusc h *et al.,* (2010)	Health-related quality of life, psychosocial strains, and coping in parents of children with chronic renal failure	Pediatr Nephrol, 225: 1477–1485.	Cross-sectional	195 parents	questionnaire for psychosocial strains, coping strategies, and Health-related quality of life (HRQOL)
Zelmer J. (2007).	The economic burden of end-stage renal disease in Canada.	Kidney International, 72; 1122–1129.	Prevalence-based approach/ incident-based human capital approach	Not stated	Not stated

Table 1: contd….

Ziegert K. et al., (2006)	Health in everyday life among spouses of haemodialysis patients: a content analysis.	Scandinavian Journal of Caring Sciences, 20(2): 223–228.	Qualitative/ Interviews	13 caregivers	Not stated

CONCLUSIONS

The literature to date presents a variety of outcomes. In most areas surveyed, especially those that concerned the more extensive studies (quality of life, depression and burden), some authors found that there was a significant impact on caregivers, but others failed to do so (Belasco *et al.*, 2006; Parlevliet *et al.*, 2012; Arechabala *et al.*, 2011; Belasco, 2002; Çelik *et al.*, 2012; Klak *et al.*, 2008), but others failed to do so (Byers *et al.*, 2011; Asti *et al.*, 2006; Wicks *et al.*, 1997; Harris *et al.*, 2000; Tzitzikos, 2010).

Caregivers of dialysis patients experience in their daily lives several stressors, which act aggregately and can trigger a host of negative emotions and events, with implications on their quality of life, health (particularly mental health), and also on the care of the patient. Several factors have been recorded as stressors: time devoted in care, financial affairs, uncertainty about the future and the disease progression (especially when the patients are children), lack of support or assistance to the caregiver, and the responsibilities of the treatment, especially in the case of home therapy (Beanlands *et al.*, 2005). However, the most determinant factor is the patient's current health status, because it directly affects all the previous factors. Patients with high co-morbidity and reduced functionality have 'de facto' more care needs that require extra time and effort from the side of caregiver, who is often pushed to his/her limits. Conversely, good health status obviously provides greater autonomy and allows for better communication, more positive relationship between patient and caregiver, while it has also a beneficial effect on their psychology (Wicks *et al.*, 1997).

The environment that both patients and caregivers live in, establishes a framework of possibilities or limitations, facilitating or hindering respectively, the satisfaction of existing needs. In addition, other factors such as cultural characteristics, social and religious beliefs related to one's worldview and the role of the individual in society, can sometimes strengthen the caregivers in their work and some other times oppress them (Cukor *et al.*, 2007).

Thus, the differentiation in the results of studies regarding caregivers should be interpreted in the light of the presence of these factors which shape the experiences of caregivers and determine their needs. Needs that can not be documented adequately by the existing studies, but can be detected mainly in the fields of support and information.

When the caregiver has adequate information, understands the patient's condition, the treatment requirements and the role of care, he/she can work with less stress and greater efficiency.

On the other hand, it is argued that the most frequent and perhaps the greater need that caregivers have, is the one for help. Researchers agree on the value of the assistance that may be offered to caregivers in order for them to lift the burden of care giving more easily (Byers *et al.*, 2011). This kind of help is multidimensional and can be provided either by members of the immediate environment of the caregiver, or by health professionals, and includes the daily tasks to be done, and the necessary psychosocial support. In addition, help to caregivers should certainly include the important parameter of time. It has been shown that the need for personal time can have a catalytic effect on the caregiver's mental balance.

After all, there is a question which usually arises in the beginning: Excluding other factors, can chronic renal failure as a disease and dialysis as a therapy process, cause a burden to caregivers, or not?

Relevant studies showing little or no burden in caregivers, do not give the answer, but just pose the question.

Thus, there are issues that were not possible to be adequately answered here. The identification of the needs could be made by instruments already available, but they do not seem to have been used for caregivers of dialysis patients. Obviously, more data are required in order to understand the impact of care on several aspects of caregivers' life, something that future research could contribute.

But, as we refer to matters related to human psyche, it should be remembered that often, in term vision prevails a subjective view which aptly attributed in the following saying of the stoic philosopher Epictetus:

"Men are disturbed not by the things which happen, but by the opinions about the things", something that applies to all aspects of human activity.

ACKNOWLEDGEMENTS

None declared

CONFLICT OF INTEREST

None declared.

REFERENCES

Aldridge, M.D. (2008). How do families adjust to having a child with chronic kidney failure? A systematic review. Nephrol Nurs J, 35(2): 157-162.

Alvarez-Ude, F., Valdés, C., Estébanez, C., Rebollo, P. (2004) Health-related quality of life of family caregivers of dialysis patients. J Nephrol, 17(6), 841–850.

American Association of Kidney Patients (2012). http://www.aakp.org/ aakplibrary/what-do-caregivers-need/index.cfm, Retrieved: 10-11-2012.

Arechabala, M.C., Catoni, M. I., Palma, E., Barrios, S. (2011). Depression and self-perceived burden of care by hemodialysis patients and their caregivers. Rev Panam Salud Publica, 30(1): 74-79. Available from: http://www.scielosp.org/scielo.php?script=sci arttext&pid=S1020-49892011000700011&lng=en.

Asti, T., Kara, M., Ipek, G., Erci, B. (2006).The experiences of loneliness, depression, and social support of Turkish patients with continuous ambulatory peritoneal dialysis and their caregivers. J Clin Nurs 15:490-497.

Belasco, A., Sesso R. (2002). Burden and quality of life of caregivers for hemodialysis patients, American Journal of Kidney Diseases, 39 (4): 805-812.

Belasco, A., Barbosa, D., Bettencourt, A., Diccini, S., Sesso, R., (2006). Quality of life of family caregivers of elderly patients on hemodialysis and peritoneal dialysis. Am J Kidney Dis; 48: 955-963.

Beanlands, H., Horsburgh, ME., Fox, S., Howe, A., Locking-Cusolito, H., Pare, K., Thrasher, C. (2005). Caregiving by family and friends of adults receiving dialysis. Nephrol Nurs J; 32:

621–631. Blogg, A. & Hyde, C. (2008) The experience of spouses caring for a person on home haemodialysis: an ethnography. Ren Soc Aust J 4(3) 75-80.

Byers, D., Mona, N., Beard, T. (2011). Depressive symptoms and health promotion behaviors of African-American women who are family caregivers of hemodialysis recipients, Nephrology Nursing Journal, v.38, no.5, Sept-Oct, p. 425(7).

Cantor, MH. (1983). Strain among caregivers. A study of the experiences in the United States. Gerontologist, 23: 597–618.

Celik G., Annagur B.B., Yilmaz M., Demir T., Kara F. (2012). Are sleep and life quality of family caregivers affected as much as those of hemodialysis patients? General Hospital Psychiatry, 34(5):518-524.

Cukor, D., Cohen, S., Peterson, R., Kimmel, P. (2007). Psychosocial Aspects of Chronic Disease: ESRD as a Paradigmatic Illness, JASN, 18: 3042-3055.

Fan SL Sathick I, McKitty K, Punzalan S(2008) Quality of life of caregivers and patients on peritoneal dialysis. Nephrol. Dial. Transplant. (23(5): 1713-1719.

Ferrario SR, Zotti AM, Baroni A, Cavagnino A, Fornara R. (2002). Emotional reactions and practical problems of the caregivers of hemodialysed patients. J Nephrol., 15(1):54-60.

Garces, J., Rodenas, F., Sanjose, V., (2003). Towards a new welfare state: the social sustainability principle and health care strategies. Health Policy 65, 201–215.

Harris, T.T., Thomas, C.M., Wicks, M.N., Faulkner, M.S., Hathaway, D.K. (2000). Subjective burden in young and older African-American caregivers of patients with end stage renal disease awaiting transplant. Nephrol Nurs J., 27(4):383-91, 355; discussion 392, 405.

Kimmel, P. (2000). Psychosocial factors in adult end-stage renal disease patients treated with hemodialysis: Correlates and outcomes, American Journal of Kidney Diseases, 35(4):132–140.

Klak R., Rymaszewska J., Watorek E., Waclaw W., Penar J., Krajewska M., Madziarska K., Klinger M., (2008). Exhaustion of caregivers of patients on maintenance haemodialysis. Nephrol Dial Transplant ; 23:4086.

Luk W.S.-C. (2002). The home care experience as perceived by the caregivers of Chinese dialysis patients. International Journal of Nursing Studies, 39 (3), 269-277.

Matsuu, K., Washio, M., Arai, Y., Higashi, H., Saku, Y., Tokunaga, S., Ide, S. (2001). Depression among caregivers of elderly patients on chronic hemodialysis. Fukuoka igaku zasshi, 92:319–25.

Mayeroff, M. (1971). On caring. Harper Perennial: New York.

McKenna AM, Keating LE, Vigneux A, Stevens S, Williams A, Geary DF.(2006) Quality of life in children with chronic kidney disease-patient and caregiver assessments. Nephrol Dial Transplant, 21(7):1899-1905.

Molumphy, S., Sporakowski, M. (1984). The Family Stress of Hemodialysis, Family Relations, 33(1):33-39.

Montgomery, R.J.V., Gonyea, J.G., & Hooyman, N.R. (1985). Caregiving and the experience of subjective and objective burden. Family Relations, 34, 19-6.

National Alliance for Caregiving in collaboration with AARP. (2009). Caregiving in the U.S.2009. Retrivent on 5th June 2012, from http://www.caregiving.org/data/Caregiving in the US 2009 full report.pdf

Newacheck, P.W. & Kim, S.E. (2005). A National Profile of Health Care Utilization and Expenditures for Children With Special Health Care Needs. Archives of Pediatric and Adolescent Medicine, 159, 10-17.

Oxford Dictionaries. (2012). Care. Retrived on: 30th July 2012, from: http://oxforddictionaries.com

Parlevliet, JL, Buurman, BM, Hodac Pannekeet, MM, Boeschoten, EM, Ten Brinke, L, Hamaker, ME., van Munster., BC., de Rooij, SE. (2012). Systematic comprehensive geriatric assessment in elderly patients on chronic dialysis: a cross-sectional comparative and feasibility study. BMC Nephrol. 30, 13(1), 30.

Pelletier-Hibbert, M., Sohi P.(2001). Sources of uncertainty and coping strategies used by family members of individuals living with end stage renal disease. Nephrol Nurs J., 28(4):411-7, 419; discussion 418-9.

Piira, T., Chow, J., Suranyi, M. (2002) The role of cognitive factors in the adjustment of home dialysis carers. Psychology Health, 17:313-322.

Rau-Foster M. (2001). The dialysis facility's rights, responsibilities, and duties when there is conflict with family members, Nephrol News Issues, 15(5):12-4.

Rioux, J.-P., Narayanan, R. and Chan, C. T. (2012), Caregiver burden among nocturnal home hemodialysis patients. Hemodialysis International. doi: 10.1111/j.1542-4758.

Schulz, R., Beach, SR. Caregiving as a Risk Factor for Mortality: The Caregiver Health Effects Study. JAMA. 1999;282(23):2215-2219.

Shimoyama, S., Hirakawa, O., Yahiro, K., Mizumach,i T., Schreine,r A., Kakuma, T. (2003). Health-related quality of life and caregiver burden among peritoneal dialysis patients and their family caregivers in Japan. Perit Dial Int., 23 Suppl 2:S200-5.

Suri, R., Larive, B., Garg, A., Hall, Y., Pierratos, A., Chertow, G., Gorodetskeya, I., Kliger, A., and for the FHN Study Group, (2011). Burden on caregivers as perceived by hemodialysis patients in the Frequent Hemodialysis Network (FHN) trials Nephrol. Dial. Transplant. 26(7): 2316-2322.

Theofilou, P. (2011). Depression and anxiety in patients with chronic renal failure: the effect of sociodemographic characteristics. International Journal of Nephrology, 2011, 1-6.

Theofilou, P. (2012). Sexual functioning in Chronic Kidney Disease: The association with depression and anxiety. Hemodialysis International, 16, 76-81.

Theofilou, P. (2012a). Self - esteem in Greek dialysis patients: The contribution of health locus of control. Iranian Journal of Kidney Diseases, 6, 136-140.

Theofilou, P. (2012b). The effect of sociodemographic features and beliefs about medicines on adherence to chronic kidney disease treatment. Journal of Clinical Research & Bioethics, 3(2), 1-5.

Theofilou, P., Synodinou, C., Panagiotaki H. (2013). Undergoing Haemodialysis - A qualitative study to investigate the lived experiences of patients. Europe's Journal of Psychology, 9, 19-32.

Theofilou, P. (2012c). Self - reported functional status: an important predictor of mental health outcomes among chronic dialysis patients. European Journal of Psychological Assessment, DOI 10.1027/1015-5759/a000155.

Tong, A., Lowe, A., Sainsbury, P., Craig, J.C. (2010).Parental perspectives on caring for a child with chronic kidney disease: an in-depth interview study. Child Care Health Dev, 36(4):549-57.

Tsai, T.C., Liu, S.I., Tsai, J.D., Chou, L.H. (2006). Psychosocial effects on caregivers for children on chronic peritoneal dialysis. Kidney Int.,70(11):1983-7.

Tzitzikos, G. (2010). Psychological features of caregivers of dialysis patients, Unpublished master's thesis, University of Thessaly, Greece.

U S Renal Data System, USRDS 2011 Annual Data Report (2011). Atlas of Chronic Kidney Disease and End-Stage Renal Disease in the United States, National Institutes of Health, National Institute of Diabetes and Digestive and Kidney Diseases, Bethesda, MD.

Van Manen M.(2000). Moral Language and pedagogical experience. Journal of Curriculum Studies, 32(2), 315-327.

Wagner, CD. (1996). Family needs of chronic hemodialysis patients: a comparison of perceptions of nurses and families. ANNA J.,23(1):19-26.

Watson, A. R. (1997). Stress and Burden of Care in Families with Children Commencing Renal Replacement Therapy. Adv Perit Dial, 13:300-4.

White, Y., Grenye,r B.F.(1999). The biopsychosocial impact of end-stage renal disease: the experience of dialysis patients and their partners. J Adv Nurs. 30(6):1312-20.

Wicks, M.N., Milstead, E.J., Hathaway, D.K., Cetingok, M. (1997). Subjective burden and quality of life in family caregivers of patients with end stage renal disease. ANNA J, 24:527-528, 531-538.

Wiedebusch, S., Konrad, M., Foppe, H., Reichwald-Klugger, E., Schaefer, F., Schreiber, V., Muthny, F.A. (2010) Health-related quality of life, psychosocial strains, and coping in parents of children with chronic renal failure. Pediatr Nephrol. 225:1477–1485.

Zarit, S.H., (2002). Caregiver's burden. In: Andrieu, S., Aquino, J.P. (Eds.), Family and Professional Caregivers: Findings Lead to Action(pp. 20–24). Paris: Serdi Edition and Fondation Mederic Alzheimer.

Ziegert, K., Fridlund, B., Lidell, E. (2006). Health in everyday life among spouses of haemodialysis patients: a content analysis. Scand J Caring Sci., 20(2):223-8.

CHAPTER 10

Stress Management, Loss and Grief in Renal Nurses

Sofia Zyga[1,*], Maria Malliarou[2], Maria Athanasopoulou[2] and Athena Kalokairinou[2]

[1]*Nursing Department, University of Peloponnese, Greece and* [2]*Nursing Department, University of Athens, Greece*

Abstract: In this chapter, we address the relationship between loss and grief that renal nurses experience and stress management. Renal nurses provide care across the life span and health continuum, including acute and chronic care to patients with kidney disease. They are involved in health promotion, illness prevention, the management of acute, chronic and terminally ill care and rehabilitation. The nurses also have to deal with sudden or unexpected death. The degree of nurses' grief as a reaction to patient death may vary in intensity. This variation may be influenced by several factors present within the nurse him/herself and the nurse–patient relationship. Due to the demands of their profession, nurses may have to suppress their grief to respond to duty's call. This prevents them from undergoing the normal grieving process, which results to a range of consequences from burnout to potentially harmful addictions. Nurse educators have identified that historically nurses have not been prepared to care for dying patients. This lack of education has been reflected in the level and quality of terminally ill care provided to patients'.

Keywords: Stress, death, loss, grief, management, nursing, haemodialysis, Renal nurses, staff, end of life, caring, peritoneal nurses, terminally ill patients, professionals, post graduate students, researchers, academicians.

STRESS MANAGEMENT, LOSS AND GRIEF IN RENAL NURSES

Nursing has been acknowledged as a very competitive working field that causes great stress to nurses. According to McVicar (2003) workload, leadership/management style, professional conflict and emotional cost of caring have been the main sources of distress for nurses for many years, but there is disagreement as to the magnitude of their impact. As Nursing is a profession that requires a high level of skill, team working in a variety of situations, provision of

*Address correspondence to Sofia Zyga:** Nursing Department, University of Peloponnese, Greece; Tel: 0030 2731089714; Fax: 00302731089721; E-mails: zygas@uop.gr; zygas@spa.forthnet.gr

Paraskevi Theofilou (Ed)

24-hour delivery of care, and input of what is often referred to as 'emotional labour' provides a wide range of potential workplace stressors (Phillips, 1996).

Nursing in haemodialysis units has been well established since 1960s, however nurse have been involved in caring for patients with identifiable renal failure since the early part of the 20th century (Hoffart, 1989). As renal failure was thought to be a terminal disease till the latter part of the century, the concept that renal nursing is a form of palliative care was a reality (Bevan, 1998). One of the major sources of stress is dealing with death and dying, grief and experience of loss. Many researchers have examined the prevalence of stress among different hospital environments and argued that coronary or intensive care nurses are presumably those that experience more stress but nursing literature review has proven that there are other specific wards where their working conditions create a great amount of stress in their personnel (Malliarou, Moustaka, Constantinidis, 2009; Malliarou, Sarafis, Moustaka, Kouvela, Constantinidis, 2010; Zyga, Malliarou, Lavdaniti, Athanasopoulou, Sarafis, 2011). To be more precise some of them are chronic kidney disease clinics, haemodialysis and peritoneal dialysis clinics, acute care nephrology wards and kidney and kidney/pancreas transplant wards and clinics. Those settings are highly demanding and nurses have to deal with death often. Causes of stress in the haemodialysis environment can be related to work colleagues (Munthy, 1989; Wellard, 1992; Lewis, Bonner, Campbell, Cooper, Willard, 1994; Klersy *et al.*, 2007), patient issues (Munthy, 1989; Brokalaki *et al.*, 2001), powerlessness (Wellard, 1992; Brokalaki *et al.*, 2001), isolation (Wellard, 1992), lack of staff support (Lewis *et al.*, 1994), personal stress (Lewis *et al.*, 1994; Klersy *et al.*, 2007) and workload (Lewis *et al.*, 1994; Brokalaki *et al.*, 2001).

Renal Nurses develop a close relationship with their patients because they may care them for years but also because they see them through many personal problems and/or triumphs, *e.g.,* birth of a child, transplantation. Approximately 15 million people worldwide are kept alive by renal dialysis (Noble, Kelly, Rawlings-Anderson, Meyer, 2007). The nephrology practice setting can be a highly emotional workplace due to the length of time the patient can be receiving care. Patients are increasingly elderly with increasing numbers of co-morbidities. Some may not be suitable for dialysis, some will choose to withdraw from treatment after a period of time and some will reach the end of their lives while still on dialysis (Ho, Barbero, Hidalgo, Camps, 2010). Renal nursing is characterized by frequent, ongoing contact with patients who have complex care requirements due to chronic kidney disease and who often have multiple concurrent illnesses; this contact is often over a number of years, occasionally decades. Work in dialysis units involves intensive and long-term contact with patients who are often frustrated or depressive, as well as confrontation with suffering and death, staff cuts and dealing with ever developing highly modern technologies (Richmond, 1986; Munthy, 1989; Anderson, Torres, Bitter, Anderson, Briefel, 1999; Brokalaki *et al.*, 2001; Kotzabassaki, Parissopoulos, 2003; Bogatz, Colasanto, Sweeney, 2005; Böhmert, Kuhnert, Nienhaus, 2011). Renal nurses have to deal either with sudden or unexpected death. Grief refers to the nurse's subjective response to the death of the patient he/she has handled. As healthcare providers who are in close contact with dying patients, nurses are vulnerable to the experience of grief (Zyga *et al.*, 2011).

In dealing with a profession as stressful as nursing, hospital managements might consider ways of reducing all major sources of stress. In some cases this will mean introducing stress management programs to help alleviate problems associated with unavoidable stressors such as dealing with death and dying patients (Patrick, Tyler, Cunningham, 1991). "There is a consensus that patient death and the subsequent grief experienced by health professionals is a significant issue and the importance of addressing must be recognized" (Macaulay, 2005). The aim of this literature review is to address the relationship between loss and grief that renal nurses experience and stress management.

STRESSFUL FACTORS IN RENAL NURSES

Stress influences all human dimensions of the individual (bodily, sentimental, mental, social and cognitive). The perception of stress as well as the reactions in this are individualised and differ not only from individual to individual but also from a time period into another in the same individual. A stressful factor is anything that makes the person experience stress. The factors that cause stress can either be from internal factors or external factors (Edwards *et al.*, 2006). Stress relates both to an individual's perception of the demands being made on them and to their perception of their capability to meet those demands. A mismatch will trigger a stress response (Clancy & McVicar, 2002). Nurses are one of the groups who can be under heavy stress at all times since they work with sick people as well as their worried families (International Council of Nurses, 2007). Renal Nurses not only form relationships with their patients and their patients' significant others but they will become familiar with the progression of the patient's illness (Binkley, 1999) recognizes that renal nurse can experience a range of different emotions when trying to deal with the dying patient. It is of great importance for the nurses who are caring for the chronic renal patients, transplanted patients, or those who are waiting for a transplant to identify their feelings about death (Kübler-Ross, 1969) has directed her efforts towards helping the health professionals understand the psychological stages of dying and their reactions to this overwhelming phenomenon. The frequency of contact with dying patients, the age of the dying patient have been recognized among the important stressors for renal nurses (Gow & Williams, 1977).

According to French (1973), the stress results from the point when the individual does not has the essential capabilities, dexterities or resources in order to satisfy the requirements that come from the working environment. The pressure that a person can experience in combination with his work it is connected with the limited harmonisation of himself with his working environment. The smaller the adaptation of the individual in the working place is, the bigger is the probability of decreased productivity, but also health problems.

The stress can emanate from:

- *The professional of health himself:* demographic characteristics (age, sex, nationality, education, previous experience, place of work), characteristics of personality (motives, expectations, ways of managing stress), previous experiences (professional or personal nature) (Papadatou, Papazoglou, Bellali, & Petraki, 1999)

- *The hospital environment of work:* conditions of work (nature of work, contact with pain and death, duties of personal care of the patient, unpleasant natural environment), organisational and administrative subjects (pressure and schedule of work, way of administration, wages, ambiguity of roles and duties) and fellowship relations (problems of collaboration and communication, lack of support) (Papadatou *et al.*, 1999).

- *The contact with ill and his relatives:* the nature of the illness (seriousness, lasting for a long time, threat of death), relations with the ill and the relatives (passive attitude or the patient's attitude of dependence, negative criticism, increased requirements and lack of recognition) (Wilson, 1996; Antoniou, 1999; Papadatou, *et al.*, 1999; Demerouti, Bakker, Nachreiner, & Schaufeli, 2000).

HSE (Health and Safety Executive, 2004) as part of their overall strategy has developed some clear guidance on stress management standards for work-related stress, launched in November 2004, encouraging organizations to take preventative measures through a risk assessment, which consists of organizations comparing themselves against:

- Demand – being able to cope with the demand of the job.

- Control – having an adequate say over how work is done.

- Support – having adequate support from colleagues and superiors.

- Roles – understanding roles and responsibilities.

- Relationships – not being subjected to unacceptable behaviors.

- Change – being involved in any organization changes.

Smith and Gray (2001) point out that new learning pattern in patient care are required to enable nurses to cope better with the emotional demands of their work. Constructive clinical supervision, mentorship, underpinned by an effective leadership style, will have a significant role to play here, especially for newly qualified nurses (Gerrish, 2000; Charnley, 1999).

RENAL NURSES AND DEATH

Research has shown that nurses play an important role in providing care and treatment for patients on the edge of life, and that this particular care situation puts heavy demands on nurses Hall (Hall, 2004).

Patients with chronic kidney disease may decline renal replacement therapy, withdraw from dialysis or may approach death while still receiving renal replacement therapy (Zyga *et al.*, 2011). Nurses' who work with the dying and their bereaved relatives are regularly brought face to face with their own mortality and also that of their family. This self-awareness can lead to a higher level of stress than perhaps the nurse can deal with (Spencer, 1994). Pearlman *et al.*, (1969) studied the attitudes towards death among nursing home personnel. They found that the staff with most experience had the most difficulty in discussing death with dying patients. Dunn *et al.*, (2005) added to the factors affecting nurses' reactions towards death, the nursing experience, while Parkes (Hall, 2004) related age, coping ability, support system, and how the bereaved perceived the loss. According to Kübler-Ross (1969), the fear of death could be reduced by improving interpersonal communication with all patients: 'If we could combine the teachings of the new scientific and technical achievements with equal emphasis on interpersonal human relationships we would indeed make progress (Kübler-Ross, 1969).

Caring of a life-threatening illness may in certain cases trigger unmanageable reactions (Wrenn, 1998). The process of death, the loss of human life and the period between life and death are the biggest challenges that renal nurses have to face in their duties. Various scientific, social and religious theories try to give answers to multidimensional relationship between patients with a life-threatening illness and nurse (Katsimigas, Maragouti, Spiliopoulou, & Gika, 2007). Watson's theory about the factors that promote the growth of a helping-trust relationship and assistance with meeting patients' needs (Tomey & Alligood, 2006) requires the nurse to commit in true care for the patient, respect human dignity and patients decisions (Watson, 1988). A nurse must examine his/her own attitudes toward death before being able to truly care for the dying patient. Nurses can change the way end-of-life care is delivered by becoming aware of these attitudes and striving to recognize death as a natural part of life (Ciccarello, 2003).

In order to provide appropriate end of-life care, nurses must overcome their anxiety and create a caring environment in which the therapeutic process of nursing can occur (Mitchell *et al.,* 2006). Nurses must not forget cultural values and practices regarding patient death and dying. Research has shown that nurses often fail to recognize that grieving and mourning are influenced by different cultures (Ciccarello, 2003; Zyga *et al.*, 2011). Being culturally aware and knowledgeable can ease the end-of-life process.

CONCLUSIONS

Nurses are present at both the beginning and the end of life, and play a key role in caring for dying patients. That role is seen as one of the most stressful facets of nursing (Hopkinson , Hallett, & Luker, 2005). Severe distress is closely linked to staff absenteeism, poor staff retention, and ill-health (Healy & McKay, 1999; McGowan, 2001; Shader, Broome, West, & Nash, 2001). It is especially burdensome for the nurse to communicate with the dying patient about death and end-of-life issues (Dean, 1998; Sasahara, Miyashita, Kawa, & Kazuma, 2003). Death anxiety is also an important factor when caring for terminally ill or dying patients. A mentor could alleviate stress for nurses who are caring for dying patients and prevent subsequent burnout. Miyashita *et al.,* (2007) conclude in their research that enhancing nursing autonomy might alleviate difficulties with communication that nurses experience when they are caring for dying patients. Educational and administrative effort to strengthen nursing autonomy is necessary.

ACKNOWLEDGEMENT

None Declared.

CONFLICT OF INTEREST

None Declared.

REFERENCES

Anderson, J. E., Torres, J. R., Bitter, D. C., Anderson, S. C. & Briefel, G. R. (1999). Role of physician's assistants in dialysis units and nephrology. American Journal of Kidney Diseases: The Official Journal of the National Kidney Foundation 33(4), 647-651.

Antoniou, A. (1999). Personal traits and professional burnout in health professional. Archives of Hellenic Medicine, 16, 20-28.

Bevan, M. T. (1998). Nursing in the dialysis unit: technological enframing and a declining art, or an imperative for caring. Journal of Advanced Nursing, 27, 730-736.

Binkley, L. (1999). Caring for renal patients during loss and bereavement. EDTA/ERCA Journal, 15(2), 45-48.NA

Bogatz, S., Colasanto, R. & Sweeney, L. (2005). Defining the impact of high patient/staff ratios on dialysis social workers. Nephrology News & Issues, 19(2), 55-60.

Böhmert, M., Kuhnert, S. & Nienhaus, A. (2011). Psychological stress and strain in dialysis staff-a systematic review. Journal of Renal Care, 37(4), 178-189.

Brokalaki, H., Matziou, V., Thanou, J., Zirogiannis, P., Dafni, U. & Papadatou, D. (2001). Job-related stress among nursing personnel in Greek dialysis units. EDTA/ERCA Journal, 27(4), 181-186.

Charnley, E. (1999). Occupational stress in the newly qualified staff nurse. Nursing Standard 13, 33–36.

Ciccarello, G. P. (2003). Strategies to improve end-of-life care in the intensive care unit. Dimensions in Critical Care Nursing, 22(5), 216-222.

Clancy, J. & McVicar, A. (2002). Physiology and Anatomy: A Homeostatic Approach, 2nd ed. Chapter 22: Stress. London: Arnold. pp. 611–633.

Dean, R. A. (1998). Occupational stress in hospice care: causes and coping strategies. American Journal of Hospice & Palliative Care, 15, 151-154.

Demerouti, E., Bakker, A., Nachreiner, F. & Schaufeli, W. (2000). A model of burnout and life satisfaction amongst nurses. Journal of Advanced Nursing, 32, 454-464.

Dunn, K. S., Otten, C. & Stephens, E. (2005). Nursing experience and the care of dying patients. Oncology Nursing Forum, 32(1), 97-104.

Edwards, D., Burnard, P., Hannigan, B., Cooper, L., Adams, J. & Juggessur, T. (2006). Clinical supervision and burnout: the influence of clinical supervision for community mental health nurses. Journal of Clinical Nursing, 15,1007–1015.

French, K. (1973). Person-role fit. Occupational Mental Health, 3, 15-20.

Gerrish, K. (2000). Still fumbling along? A comparative study of the newly qualified nurses' perception of the transition from student to qualified nurse. Journal of Advanced Nursing 32, 473– 480.

Gow, C. & Williams, I. (1977). Nurses attitudes toward death and dying: A causal interpretation. Social Science & Medicine, (II), 191-198.

Hall, EOC. (2004). A double concern: Danish grandfathers' experiences when a small grandchild is critically ill. Intensive Critical Care, 20, 14–21.

Healy, C., & McKay, M. F. (1999). Identifying sources of stress and job satisfaction in the nursing environment. Australian Journal of Advanced Nursing, 17, 30–35.

Ho, T. M., Barbero E., Hidalgo, C. & Camps, C. (2010). Spanish nephrology nurses' views and attitudes towards caring for dying patients. Journal of Renal Care, 36(1), 2-8.

Hoffart, N. (1989). Nephrology nursing 1915-1970. A historical of the integration of technology and care. American Nephrology Nurses Association Journal, 16(3), 169-178.

Hopkinson, J.B., Hallett, C. E. & Luker, K. A. (2005). Everyday death: how do nurses cope with caring for dying people in hospital? International Journal of Nursing Studies, 42, 125-133.

HSE (Health and Safety Executive). (2004). Management standards for work-related stress. London: HSE. Retrieved May 22, 2012 from http//www.hse.gov.uk/stress/standards.

International Council of Nurses (2007). Nurses need stress management. Retrieved June 14, 2012 from www.stressfreecontrol.com

Katsimigas, G., Maragouti, K., Spiliopoulou, C. & Gika, M. (2007). Nursing and theological access to death. Nosileftiki, 46(4), 441–452.

Klersy, C., Callegari, A., Martinelli, V., Vizzardi, V., Navino C., & Malberti, F. (2007). Burnout in health care providers of dialysis service in Northern Italy—a multicenter study. Nephrology. Dialysis, Transplantation, 22(8), 2283-2290.

Kotzabassaki, S., & Parissopoulos, S. (2003). Burnout in renal care professionals. EDTNA ERCA Journal, 29(4), 209-213.

Kübler-Ross, E. (1969). On death and dying. New York: Collier Books.

Lewis, S., Bonner, P., Campbell, M., Cooper, C. L. & Willard, A. (1994). Personality, stress, coping, and sense of coherence among nephrology nurses in dialysis settings. American Nephrology Nurses Journal, 21(6), 325-335.

Macaulay, J. (2005). When Patients Die: Grief amongst Health Care Professionals. The Canadian Journal of Medical Radiation Technology, 36(1), 17.

Malliarou, M., Sarafis, P., Moustaka, E., Kouvela T. & Constantinidis, T. C. (2010). Greek Registered Nurses' Job Satisfaction in Relation to Work-Related Stress. A Study on Army and Civilian RNs. Global Journal of Health Science, 2010, 2(1) 44-60.

Malliarou., M., Moustaka, E. & Constantinidis, T. C. (2009). Stress related health problems and management of occupational stress. Public Health and Health Care in Greece and Bulgaria: The Challenge of the Cross-border Collaboration. Alexandroupolis, Greece.

Mc Vicar, A. (2003). Workplace stress in nursing: a literature review. Journal of Advanced Nursing, 44(6), 633–642.

McGowan, B. (2001). Self-reported stress and its effects on nurses. Nursing Standard, 15, 33–38.

Mitchell, A. M., Sakraida, T. J., Dysart-Gale, D. & Gadmer, N. (2006). Nurses' narratives of end-of-life care. Journal of Hospice and Palliative Nursing, 8(4), 210-221.

Miyashita, M., Nakai, Y., Sasahara, T., Koyama, Y., Shimizu, Y., Tsukamoto, N. & Kawa, M. (2007). Nursing Autonomy Plays an Important Role in Nurses' Attitudes Toward Caring for Dying Patients. American Journal of Hospice & Palliative Care, 24, 202.

Munthy, F. (1989). Job strains and job satisfaction of dialysis nurses. Psychotherapy Pyschosomatics, 51(3), 150-155.

Noble, H., Kelly, D., Rawlings-Anderson, K. & Meyer, J. (2007). A concept analysis of renal supportive care: the changing world of nephrology. Journal of Advanced Nursing, 59(6), 644-653.

Papadatou, D., Papazoglou, I., Bellali, T. & Petraki, D. (1999). Mutual support among nurses who provide care to dying children illness. Crisis and Loss, 7, 37-48.

Patrick, A., Tyler D. C. & Cunningham S. E. (1991). Stress and well-being in nurses: a comparison of the public and private sectors. International Journal of Nursing Studies, 28(2), 125-130.

Pearlman, J., Stotsky, A. & Dominick, J. R. (1969). Attitudes toward death among nursing home personnel. Journal of Genetic Psychology, 114, 63-75.

Phillips, S. (1996). Labouring the emotions: Expanding the remit of nursing work? Journal of Advanced Nursing, 24(2), 139-143.

Richmond, I. J. (1986). Dialysis nurses coping with stress through a peer support group. Journal of Nephrology Nursing, 3(2), 52-54.

Sasahara, T., Miyashita, M., Kawa, M. & Kazuma, K. (2003). Difficulties encountered by nurses in the care of terminally ill cancer patients in general hospitals in Japan. Journal of Palliative Medicine, 2003, 17, 520-526.

Shader, K., Broome, M.E., West, M.E. & Nash, M. (2001). Factors influencing satisfaction and anticipated turnover for nurses in an academic medical center. Journal of Nursing Administration, 31, 210–216.

Smith, P. & Gray, B. (2001). Reassessing the concept of emotional labour in student nurse education: role of link lecturers and mentors in time of change. Nurse Education Today 21, 230–237.

Spencer, L. (1994). How do nurses deal with their own grief when a patient dies on an intensive care unit, and what help can be given to enable them to overcome their grief effectively? Journal of Advanced Nursing, 19(6), 1141-1150.

Tomey, A. M., & Alligood, M. R. (2006). Nursing theorists and their work (6th ed.). St. Louis: Mosby.

Watson, J. (1988). Nursing: human science and human care. A theory of nursing. New York: National League for Nursing.

Wellard, S. (1992). The nature of dilemmas in dialysis nurse practice. Journal of Advanced Nursing, 17, 951-958.

Wilson, A. (1996). Exhaustion syndrome in palliative care. Support Care Cancer, 4, 408-415.

Wrenn, R. (1998). The process of mourning. In Nilsen, M., Papadatou, D. Mourning in our Lives. Athens: Merimna. [In Greek].

Zyga, S., Malliarou, M., Lavdaniti, M., Athanasopoulou, M. & Sarafis, P. (2011). Greek renal nurses' attitudes towards death. Journal of Renal Care, 37(2),101-107

Send Orders of Reprints at reprints@benthamscience.net

CHAPTER 11

Treatment of Chronic Kidney Disease: A Comparative Cost Analysis of Bicarbonate Dialysis and Haemodiafiltration

Paraskevi Theofilou[1,*] and Helen Panagiotaki[2]

[1]*National School of Public Administration, Department of Health Services Administration, Athens, Greece and* [2]*"A. Fleming" General Hospital of Melissia, Melissia, Athens, Greece*

Abstract: The aim of the present paper is the economic evaluation of haemodialysis in a dialysis unit of a private clinic. Specifically, a comparative cost analysis between bicarbonate dialysis and haemodiafiltration is performed. One hundred and twenty (120) patients with end - stage kidney disease, undergoing haemodialysis participated in the study. Demographic, clinical and financial characteristics were taken from the patients' medical records. Data were collected from the financial management of the clinic regarding staff salaries, capital and technological equipment, depreciation, expenditure on fixed assets and other consumables. Values of 2007 were used and haemodialysis session was considered as the unit of cost. The total cost of haemodiafiltration predominates by about 30% of bicarbonate dialysis. This significant increase in cost is due to the additional health equipment required in this method (bags and lines of haemodiafiltration). Haemodialysis is a highly expensive method of treating patients with chronic kidney disease, as based mainly on the use of innovative technologies. Similar analyses of economic evaluation are not considered fully documented, when not taking into account the clinical superiority and not attributing it in terms of cost - effectiveness.

Keywords: Economic evaluation, cost analysis, chronic kidney disease, haemodialysis, bicarbonate dialysis, haemodiafiltration.

INTRODUCTION

In Medicine, mainly in western societies, the last decades are characterized by great achievements in the treatment of various diseases. Modern technology and especially the biotechnology industry, which has expanded significantly in the areas of pathologies treatment and medical care of patients, now offers increased

Address correspondence to Paraskevi Theofilou: National School of Public Administration, Department of Health Services Administration, Athens, Greece; Tel: +0030 6977441502, Fax: +0030 2106221435; E-mail: theofi@otenet.gr; paraskevi.theofilou@gmail.com

retention capabilities and elongation of life for major categories of chronically ill individuals, who were once left to their fate (Apostolou, 2000). Thus, longer than the survival, the way one survives, the possibility of full or partial recovery, and its evaluation, became additional medical objectives. Today's society of the western world is an aging society more than the old, resulting in the increase and prevalence of chronic diseases. As a default, a therapy that addresses chronic patients is not intended to cure but mainly to the increase in life expectancy and the maintenance of a decent quality of the rest of their lives.

It is a fact that since the late 70s, there is a continuous effort for the treatment of chronic kidney disease (CKD), resulting in more and more new dialysis machines, less costly and less tiring for the patient. Around these issues intense reflection began to grow among health economists with object to achieve the lowest possible social and economic costs in combination with efficient treatment method, so be offered for these patients the best possible quality of life (QoL).

All of the above, in developed countries, have been seriously taken into account in the formulation of health policy in patients with CKD, to result in the adoption of renal transplantation as treatment dominant method.

In our country, neither the state nor the insurers have not yet dealt with the comparative cost-benefit between alternative therapies, although large amounts are spent for this group of patients, thus dialysis in hospital remains as the basic method of treatment.

The need, therefore, to reduce cost in combination with the existence of options in every act or function that requires financial sacrifices makes economic evaluation as a necessary methodological tool, which helps specialists to make rational decisions (Kyriopoulos & Niakas, 1994). On the other hand, in the case of private investment, the application of economic evaluation in the private sector seeks to justify the selection of specific decisions, by purely economic criteria and the final profit target.

It is therefore imperative to conduct economic studies in order to record the factors that directly or indirectly affect the cost, so that research is directed towards specific measures to minimize it.

The present work through the economic evaluation for one of the two methods of dialysis, aspires to contribute to or at least to pique interest in developing further reflection and study of an alternative form of financing. Moreover, the calculation of the cost of treatment can be the starting point to perform cost - effectiveness studies, enabling benchmarking the effectiveness and efficiency of these.

MATERIAL AND METHOD

The aim of this study is the evaluation of the dialysis cost at a private clinic in 2007. The whole effort based on data of patients' records collected from the dialysis unit of the private clinic. Dialysis session was used as unit of measurement.

To estimate the cost of dialysis, cost analysis was applied, on which factors were recorded which contribute to the final cost of renal replacement treatment. In particular, to estimate each component in resource use (*e.g.,* investigations, medicines, sanitary material *etc.*), cost analysis was performed (Drummond, 1997).

One hundred and twenty (120) patients participated in the study diagnosed with end - stage kidney disease (ESKD), who were undergoing haemodialysis (HD) for the year 2007.

The dialysis unit operates six (6) days per week (Monday - Saturday) while there are twenty - one (21) dialysis stations. During 2007, a total of 18.801 haemodialysis sessions were performed. In the artificial kidney unit of the private clinic, the following two types of dialysis are performed:

➢   Haemodialysis with bicarbonate solution and bicarbonate cartridge,

➢   Haemodiafiltration (HDF) using membranes of high permeability.

Of the total dialysis sessions, which took place in 2007 (18.801), 13.161 (70%) were performed with haemodialysis with bicarbonate solution and bicarbonate cartridge, while the remaining 5.640 were performed by the method of haemodiafiltration (30%) (graph **1**).

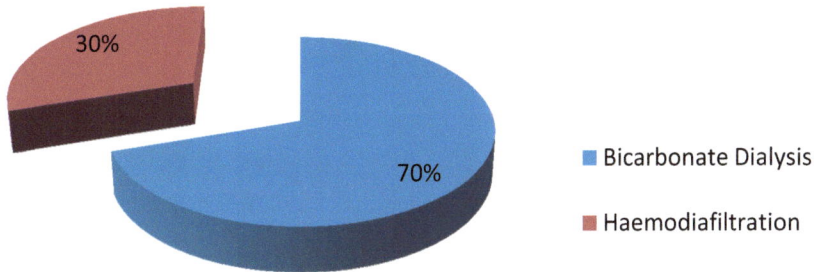

Graph 1: Sessions per method of dialysis in 2007.

As shown, in this clinic wide application of dialysis with bicarbonate solution and bicarbonate cartridge is made compared to HDF.

To calculate the cost, the following factors were studied:

- Wage costs of staff who are engaged in the dialysis unit.

- The cost of medication taken by haemodialysis patients and associated with the treatment of CKD.

- Equipment costs (purchase-depreciation-maintenance).

- The cost of building installations.

- The cost of laboratory tests.

- The cost of medical supplies (general and special) used to carry a dialysis session, depending on the type of dialysis.

- The cost of support services and other consumables (water, telephone, heating, *etc.*).

RESULTS

In Table **1**, the total session cost is presented for each type of dialysis. Specifically, the total session cost amounts to 329.61€ for dialysis with cartridge and bicarbonate solution. The greater part of the session costs occupy drugs with 46% because erythropoietin obtained by patients is too expensive. Here is the health material with 29%, since the materials used (*e.g.,* filters) are also very expensive and then staff salaries at the rate of 13% of the total cost (graph **2**).

On the other hand, the total session cost amounts to 421.67€ for dialysis with the method of haemodiafiltration (Table **1**).

This increase in 30% about compared to the cartridge dialysis and bicarbonate solution is due to the additional materials used in this method which are extremely expensive (bags and lines of haemodiafiltration). Therefore, in haemodiafiltration the share of medical supplies is increased and amounts to 45% of the total cost of dialysis followed by the cost of medicines by 36% and the staff salaries by 10% (graph **3**).

In Table **2**, the cost per patient is presented for 2007, who follows a bicarbonate dialysis program. The total cost is 51.419.16€.

Most part occupies medication with 46%. Here is the health material with 29% and then staff salaries with rate 13% of the total cost.

Regarding the annual cost per patient, who follows dialysis program with the method of haemodiafiltration, this amounts to 65.780.52€ for 2007 (Table **3**).

In haemodiafiltration the share of medical supplies is increased and amounts to 45% of the total dialysis cost per patient followed by the cost of medicines by 36% and of staff salaries by 10%.

Table 1: Total cost session per each type of dialysis.

Distribution of Operating Costs	HD with Bicarbonate	Haemodiafiltration
Staff salaries	43.00	43.00
Medicines	151.87	151.87
Equipment (maintenance – depreciation)	21.46	21.46
Buildings 5.32	5.32	
Laboratory tests	7.53	7.53
Health equipment 97.08	189.14	
Support services & other consumables	3.35	3.35
TOTAL	329.61€	421.67€

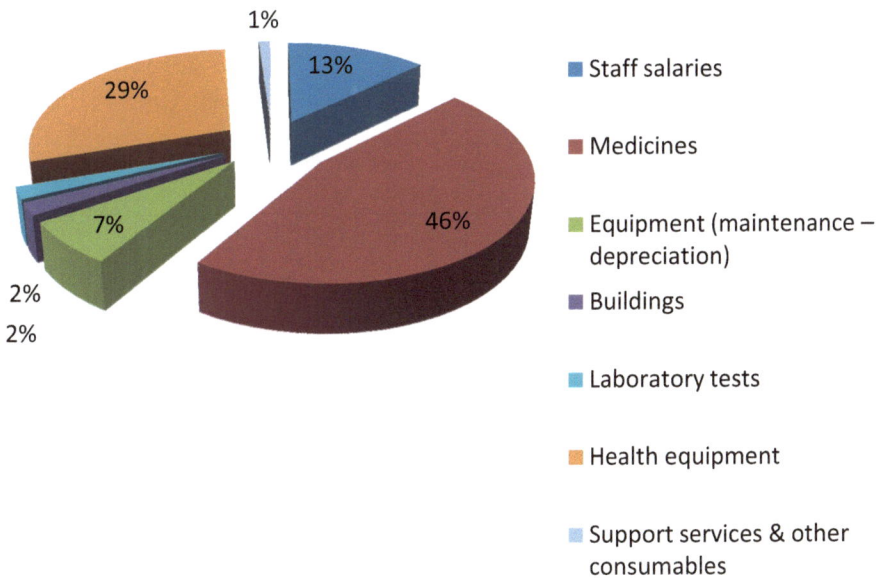

Graph 2: Total cost of a session with bicarbonate dialysis.

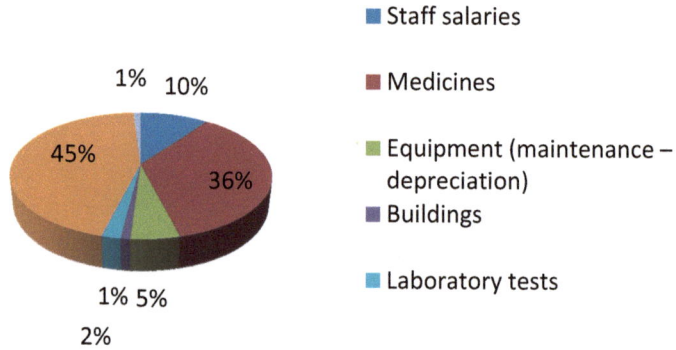

Graph 3: Total cost of a session with haemodiafiltration.

Table 2: Annual costs per patient (dialysis with cartridge and bicarbonate solution).

Distribution of Operating Costs	Cost per Patient (in €)	% (Percentage)
Staff salaries	6708.00	13%
Medicines	23691.72	46%
Equipment (maintenance – depreciation)	3347.76	7%
Buildings	829.92	2%
Laboratory tests	1174.68	2%
Health equipment	15144.48	29%
Support services & other consumables	522.60	1%
TOTAL	51.419.16	100%

Table 3: Annual costs per patient (dialysis with the method of haemodiafiltration).

Distribution of Operating Costs	Cost per Patient (in €)	% (Percentage)
Staff salaries	6708.00	10%
Medicines	23691.72	36%
Equipment (maintenance – depreciation)	3347.76	5%
Buildings	829.92	1%
Laboratory tests	1174.68	2%
Health equipment	29505.84	45%
Support services & other consumables	522.60	1%
TOTAL	65780.52	100%

DISCUSSION

It is undeniable that better knowledge on efficiency and cost of different health interventions will allow the achievement of the final goal which is the correct and cost effective management of the disease (Liaropoulos, 1996α). Indispensable tool in this process are the socio-economic evaluation studies, which are based on the results of the medical work to list either the cost of the project or compare alternative therapeutic interventions that have different costs and consequences (Kyriopoulos & Niakas, 1994; Geitona, 1996).

The dialysis is a very expensive treatment of ESKD patients, since it is based mainly on the use of innovative technologies. The cost increases with the use of new methods of dialysis, as the haemodiafiltration examined. The more expensive material used is increasing by 30% the cost in comparison to cartridge dialysis and bicarbonate solution.

Medications are the most important factor in shaping the cost after occupying the 46% of the overall cost of dialysis with bicarbonate because of erythropoietin which is a very expensive. Additionally, one of the key factors behind the high cost is the health equipment, which in dialysis with bicarbonate solution and cartridge covers 29% of the total method cost. This contributes to the high cost of filters that are used only once for each session. The payroll is the third important determinant of the final cost with turnout 13% of the total cost of dialysis with cartridge and bicarbonate solution.

Passing to dialysis with the method of haemodiafiltration, the main factors that shape the overall cost are the same. However, the rates change due to the expensive materials used in this method, thereby increasing the rate of medical supplies (45% from 29% with cartridge and bicarbonate solution) at the total cost of dialysis by this method.

The results of the present study regarding the comparative evaluation of these two methods agree with the results of similar studies (Tediosi *et al.*, 2001; Piccoli *et al.*, 1997; Rodriguez-Carmona *et al.*, 1996), whereby the dialysis method with haemodiafiltration is more expensive compared to dialysis with bicarbonate.

Therefore, it becomes clear that the record of the dialysis cost enables us on the one side to focus on the factors, which form the total cost (if this method is the most widespread in Greece), so that we can help to control and the other for comparison, regarding the cost, to alternative therapies of ESKD, *i.e.,* peritoneal dialysis and kidney transplantation.

This also shows and a series of investigations, that haemodialysis is more expensive from peritoneal dialysis by 20% (Kontodimopoulos *et al.*, 2005; Rozenbaum *et al.*, 1985; Goeree *et al.*, 1995; Rodriguez-Carmona *et al.*, 1996), 60% more expensive, in other investigations, with sodium bicarbonate and twice with the method of haemodiafiltration (Tediosi *et al.*, 2001). This is based on the fact that the treatment is done in the hospital thereby generating significant personnel costs in contrast to peritoneal dialysis performed at home. In this case, however, the cost of educating a patient to apply the same treatment at home should be taken into consideration (Kontodimopoulos *et al.*, 2005).

The cost per patient for 2007 amounts to 51.419.16 Euros for haemodialysis with bicarbonate. On the other hand, the annual cost per patient amounts to 65.780.52 Euros for haemodiafiltration. The difference is explained, as mentioned earlier, because of more expensive materials, used in haemodialysis by the method of haemodiafiltration.

So, given the ever increasing cost of tackling ESKD and the scarcity of resources, data from such studies may prove useful in decision making for selection methods of ESKD treatment. This possibility must build our country and in this sense, great weight must be given to the use of economic evaluation techniques often applied instead of making tacit decisions, where choices and the very important matter of resource allocation is based on standard medical practices and historical data without taking into account the current needs and of course the preferences and patients' QoL. Under these conditions, *i.e.,* avoiding the application of scientific methods of evaluation on one hand, it is not possible to rationalize the allocation of resources and cost effectiveness of health programs and also equality and social justice problems may be created because the misuse of resources may lead to exclusion of new health services in important segments of population.

ACKNOWLEDGEMENT

None Declared.

CONFLICT OF INTEREST

None Declared.

REFERENCES

Apostolou Th. (2000). Quality of Life: A neglected parameter of evaluation of therapeutic decisions. Greek Nephrology. 12(1): 28-33.

Geitona M. (1996). Health Policy and Health Economics. Athens: Exantas.

Drummond M, O' Brien B, Stoddart G, & Torrance G. (1997). Methods of health programmes economic evaluation. Athens: Kritiki.

Goeree R, Manalich J, Grootendorst P, Beecroft ML, & Churchill DN. (1995). Cost analysis of dialysis treatments for end-stage renal disease. Clin Invest Med, 18: 455-464.

Kontodimopoulos N, Niakas D, & Mylonakis J. (2005). A socio-economic comparison of haemodialysis and peritoneal dialysis in Greece. Int J Health Care Tech Manag, 6: 296-306.

Kyriopoulos I, & Niakas D. (1994). Health Policy and Health Economics Issues. Athens: Centre of Social Sciences of Health.

Liaropoulos L. (1996α). Pharmacoeconomic studies and methodological issues of cost accounting. Pharmaceutical, 9 (III): 97-105.

Piccoli G, Formica M, Mangiarotti G, Pacitti A, Piccoli GB, Bajardi P, Cavagnino A, Ghezzi P, Rangi R, Ramello A, Verzetti G, Cesano G, Quarello F, & Vercellone A. (1997). The cost of dialysis in Italy. Nephrol Dial Transplant, 12 (Suppl. 1): 33-44.

Rodriguez-Carmona A, Perez Fontan M, Bouza P, Garcia Falcon T, & Valdes F. (1996). The economic cost of dialysis: a comparison between peritoneal dialysis and in-center haemodialysis in a Spanish unit. Adv Perit Dial, 12: 93-96.

Rozenbaum AE, Pliskin JS, Barnoon S, & Chaimovitz C. (1985). Comparative study of costs and quality of life of chronic ambulatory peritoneal dialysis and haemodialysis patients in Israel. Israel Journal of Medical Sciences, 21: 335-339.

Tediosi F, Bertolini G, Parazzini F, Mecca G. & Garattini, L. (2001). Cost analysis of dialysis modalities in Italy. Health Serv Manag Res, 14: 9-17.

Send Orders of Reprints at reprints@benthamscience.net

CHAPTER 12

The Economic Burden of Dialysis Patients in Belgium: a Comparison Between Haemo and Peritoneal Dialysis

Max Dratwa[1], Anne-Marie Bogaert[2], Koen Bouman[3], Xavier Warling[4], Remi Hombrouckx[5], Mario Schurgers[6], Pierre Dupont[7], Anne Vereerstraeten[8], Guy Van Roost[9], Karin Caekelbergh[10],*, Mark Lamotte[10] and Suzanne Laplante[11]

[1]*CHU Brugmann, Brussels, Belgium;* [2]*AZ Sint Elisabeth, Zottegem, Belgium;* [3]*ZNA, Middelheim, Antwerp, Belgium;* [4]*Center Hospital Régionale Citadelle, Liège, Belgium;* [5]*AZ Zusters van Barmhartigheid, Ronse, Belgium;* [6]*AZ St. Jan, Brugge, Belgium;* [7]*CHU Tivoli, La Louvière, Belgium;* [8]*CHU André Vésale, Montigny-Le-Tilleul;* [9]*St. Jan Hospital Brussels, Belgium;* [10]*Health Economics and Outcomes Research, IMS Health, Brussels, Belgium and* [11]*Baxter Healthcare Corporation, Baxter World Trade SA/NV, Belgium*

Abstract: The number of patients on dialysis has increased by about 50% in the past decade in Belgium. This growth is expected to continue, albeit at a slower pace, due to the ageing of the population and the increased prevalence of hypertension and diabetes, two of the main causes of end-stage kidney disease. The aim of this study was to assess the economic burden (*i.e.*, dialysis procedure; hospitalizations; ambulatory care; medications; transport) to the public healthcare payer of patients undergoing dialysis in Belgium. Records of 130 Belgian patients on dialysis in 2006 were retrospectively reviewed to identify direct medical and non-medical resources used over a year. Official tariffs were used to cost the resources. Considering the prevalence of each dialysis modality in Belgium, the average cost of a dialysis patient was found to be €70,649 per year (haemodialysis: €72,350; peritoneal dialysis: €55,343). The dialysis procedure itself was the main cost driver (66% of all costs) followed by hospitalizations and ambulatory care (16% of all costs each). The dialysis procedure *per se* was 27% more expensive, while hospital and ambulatory services were respectively 28% and 45% more expensive for haemodialysis than peritoneal dialysis patients. Considering that there were 6,607 patients on dialysis in Belgium (0.06% of the Belgian population) at the end of 2006, it is estimated that the economic burden to the Belgian healthcare system was 467 million Euro or 2.45% of the healthcare budget. This study provides further evidence that home modalities, such as peritoneal dialysis, could help reduce the economic burden of dialysis on the healthcare budget.

*Address correspondence to Karin Caekelbergh:** Health Economics and Outcomes Research, IMS Health, Medialaan 38, Vilvoorde, Belgium; Tel: +32 93741233; Fax: +32 93741033; E-mail: KCaekelbergh@be.imshealth.com

Keywords: Dialysis, haemodialysis, home dialysis, peritoneal dialysis, healthcare costs, Belgium, economic burden.

INTRODUCTION

In the last decade, the prevalence of patients on renal replacement therapy (RRT) in Belgium has increased on average by 4.6% per year (European Renal Association-European Dialysis and Transplant Association (ERA-EDTA), 2009; ERA-EDTA, 2011; Kramer *et al* 2009). According to the most recent annual report of ERA-EDTA (2011) there were 12,558 patients on RRT in Belgium at the end of 2009. Of these, 6,746 (53.7%) were on hemodialysis (HD), 699 (5.6%) on peritoneal dialysis (PD) and 5,113 (40.7%) had a functioning kidney transplant (399 transplants in 2009).

There are several factors explaining this increase. The Belgian population is ageing, and diseases such as diabetes and hypertension, two important causes of renal failure, have become more prevalent. In addition, the improvements seen over the last two decades in the survival of dialysis and transplant patients have contributed to increasing the pool of prevalent patients (Kramer *et al.,* 2009).

Dialysis is an expensive treatment and although a small (0.06%) proportion of the population was on dialysis, in 2008, 1.57% (336 million €) (Cleemput *et al.,* 2010) of the total annual healthcare budget in Belgium was used for dialysis (dialysis procedure only).

The reimbursement of dialysis in Belgium is based on fixed tariffs. The dialysis centre receives a fixed amount from the public healthcare payer (Ministry of Social Affairs – MoSA) per HD session or per week of PD. This reimbursement covers the procedure *per se*, the disposables, staff and capital costs (chair, dialysis and water treatment machines, *etc.*). Hospitalizations, laboratory and diagnostic tests, medications, as well as other ambulatory care and transport are covered separately.

In general, the dialysis procedure costs are lower for PD than for HD (Just *et al.,* 2008). However, little is known about the other healthcare resources and costs dialysis patients may consume.

The aim of the current study was to assess the economic burden of patients requiring dialysis to the Belgian public healthcare payer (*e.g.*, dialysis procedure; hospitalizations, ambulatory care, medications, transport).

SUBJECTS AND METHODS

Patients on dialysis on January 1, 2006 at 9 Belgian dialysis-centers were randomly selected and their hospital records were retrospectively reviewed for direct medical and non-medical resources used during the year. The study had a pragmatic design where inclusion criteria were limited to: i) undergoing dialysis in 2006 and ii) having documented follow-up throughout the year. Similarly, exclusion criteria were limited to: i) lost to follow-up (death was not an exclusion criterion as it was a possible outcome of treatment/disease) and ii) participation into a clinical trial (to avoid any protocol-driven resource use). Each center provided a list of their patients on chronic dialysis (initials, year of birth, dialysis modality: in-center HD (ICHD), limited care HD (LCHD), home HD (HHD), continuous ambulatory PD (CAPD), automated PD (APD). The lists were pooled and a random selection of 130 patient records to be reviewed for the study was performed by IMS-Health so that an equal number of patients per dialysis modality was to be achieved (*i.e.*, 5 times 26 patients). This sample size was based on an 80%-probability of detecting a 30% difference in overall costs between the different dialysis groups with a 2-sided type I (α) error of 5%. The clinic charts were reviewed in the 4th quarter of 2007.

Information collected included the type of dialysis modality, baseline medical characteristics, frequency and number of dialysis sessions, type of vascular access, number/volume of exchanges of peritoneal dialysis, duration and reason for hospitalization, type and frequency of ambulatory care, medication and transport. The study was approved by the Ethics Committee (EC) of each participating center and informed consent was obtained.

After data collection and entry, co-morbidities were reviewed independently by two individuals with medical background and a Charlson's Comorbidity Index (CCI) score was given to each patient based on the scoring scale adapted for renal disease (Beddhu, Burns, Saul, Seddon, & Zeidel, 2000). The agreed scores were reviewed and corrected, if needed, by a nephrologist. An ANOVA test was performed to detect differences in CCI scores between dialysis subgroups. A Chi-Square test was performed to detect differences in CCI scores categories (mild: 0 to 3; moderate: 4-5; high: 6-7; very high: ≥ 8) between dialysis-subgroups. Significant differences between dialysis modalities would preclude analysis per modality and data would be pooled per technique (HD *vs.* PD) to analyze differences in costs.

Direct medical costs were calculated by multiplying resource utilization with unit costs. Unit costs were obtained from the official national tariffs (INAMI/RIZIV, 2007). In Belgium, a physician fee is paid as part of the dialysis tariff only for ICHD. For LCHD, there is no physician fee paid, while for PD, the physician receives payments for follow-up visits (usually every 6 weeks). Transport costs (direct non-medical costs) were obtained by multiplying the number of kilometers from home to the dialysis centre (times 2) by the official MoSA tariff of €0.25 per kilometer. Note that in Belgium, a large part of the transport costs are assumed by the sickness funds, the patient him/herself or a charity.

To calculate the economic burden of dialysis patients in Belgium as well as the average cost per dialysis patient, the costs observed in the study sample for each dialysis modality were multiplied by the 2006 prevalence of each dialysis modality (*i.e.,* 66% ICHD, 24% LCHD, 6% APD and 4% CAPD) (ERA-EDTA, 2009).

Differences in costs were assessed with t-tests. Multifactorial regression analyses were performed to verify how factors such as the CCI score categories, the dialysis technique, and the gender were influencing the costs. All analyses were performed in Excel except the regression analysis and ANOVA (SAS).

RESULTS

Baseline Medical Characteristics and Treatment Outcomes

Due to the time elapsed between the first and the last centre agreeing and obtaining EC approval, the randomization process for the study population could not be performed as originally planned. As a result, 48 ICHD, 39 LCHD, 26 APD and 17 CAPD were recruited (HHD: 0). Baseline characteristics are presented in Table **1**.

Table 1: Baseline characteristics of the study sample (n=130).

Parameter	APD	CAPD	All PD	ICHD	LCHD	All HD	All patients	P value
N (% of total)	26 (20.0%)	17 (13.1%)	**43 (33.1%)**	48 (36.9%)	39 * (26.2%)	**87 (66.9%)**	130 (100%)	
Male (%)	19 (73.1%)	10 (58.8%)	**29 (67.4%)**	29 (60.4%)	29 (74.4%)	**58 (66.7%)**	87 (66.9%)	0.4168†
Age (years ± SD**)	56.0 ± 18.9	69.5 ± 14.5	**61.3 ± 18.6**	70.7 ± 14.5	61.6 ± 19.7	**66.6 ± 17.6**	64.9 ± 18.0	0.0025§
Weight (kg ± SD)	72.0 ± 14.6	73.3 ± 10.8	**72.5 ± 13.1**	66.9 ± 16.0	73.1 ± 16.0	**69.6 ± 15.6**	70.5 ± 14.8	0.2015§
BMI (kg/m² ± SD)	25.0 ± 6.1	28.3 ± 3.6	**26.5 ± 5.3**	24.5 ± 5.0	26.0 ± 4.8	**25.2 ± 5.0**	25.6 ± 5.1	0.1764§
Years on dialysis	2.8 ± 2.9	1.4 ± 0.9	**2.2 ± 2.4**	3.7 ± 4.6	3.6 ± 4.3	**3.7 ± 4.4**	3.2 ± 3.9	0.1611§
Comorbidities (%):								
Cardiovascular disease	9 (34.6%)	8 (47.1%)	**17 (39.5%)**	22 (45.8%)	17 (43.6%)	**39 (44.8%)**	56 (43.1%)	0.7959†
Diabetes	5 (19.2%)	10 (58.8%)	**15 (34.9%)**	15 (31.3%)	11 (28.2%)	**26 (29.9%)**	41 (31.5%)	0.5444†
Cancer	2 (7.7%)	3 (17.6%)	**5 (11.6%)**	2 (4.2%)	4 (10.3%)	**6 (6.9%)**	11 (8.5%)	0.3651†
HIV positive	2 (7.7%)	2 (11.8%)	**4 (9.3%)**	0 (0.0%)	0 (0.0%)	**0 (0.0%)**	4 (3.1%)	0.0039¶
Other	21 (80.85)	14 (82.4%)	**35 (81.4%)**	40 (83.3%)	35 (89.7%)	**75 (86.2%)**	110 (84.6%)	0.7504†

(*Including 5 patients performing night time dialysis; ** SD: standard deviation; †Chi Square test on the 4 modalities; §ANOVA on the 4 modalities; ¶Chi Square test on HD *vs.* PD).

The main causes of renal failure in these 130 patients were diabetes (20.8%), glomerulonephritis (17.7%) and renal vascular disease (16.2%). Other causes are shown in Table **2**.

The CCI-scores differed among dialysis modalities (p=0.0152). Patients on CAPD and ICHD had higher scores. Overall, 63.1% of the patients had a score of 6 or more. This proportion was 82.4% and 77.1% for CAPD and ICHD respectively, compared with 42.3% and 51.3% for APD and LCHD respectively (p=0.0061; Table **3**). When patients were grouped by type of dialysis technique (HD or PD), the scores were not different (p=0.9435) and patients with a high or very high score accounted for 58.1% and 65.5% of PD and HD patients respectively (p=0.8243). Therefore, for cost analyses, pooling patients per dialysis technique was deemed more appropriate.

Table 2: Underlying causes of kidney disease.

	APD N=26	CAPD N=17	All PD N=43	ICHD N=48	LCHD N=39	All HD N=87	All patients N=130
Underlying cause (%)*							
Diabetes	23.1%	11.8%	**18.6%**	16.7%	28.2%	**21.8%**	20.8%
Glomerulonephritis	15.4%	17.7%	**16.3%**	20.8%	15.4%	**18.4%**	17.7%
Analgesic nephropathy	0%	0%	**0%**	4.2%	2.6%	**3.4%**	2.3%
Renal vascular disease	11.5%	17.7%	**14.0%**	18.8%	15.4%	**17.2%**	16.2%
Cystic kidney disease	7.7%	0%	**4.7%**	10.4%	10.3%	**10.3%**	8.5%
Other urologic disease	7.7%	0%	**4.7%**	6.3%	5.1%	**5.7%**	5.4%
Other cause	19.2%	47.1%	**30.2%**	18.8%	18.0%	**18.4%**	22.3%
Unknown cause	15.4%	5.9%	**11.6%**	4.2%	5.1%	**4.6%**	6.9%

(*Chi Square test on the 4 modalities, $p=0.5657$).

Table 3: Charlson's comorbidity index scores.

	APD N=26	CAPD N=17	All PD N=43	ICHD N=48	LCHD N=39	All HD N=87	All patients N=130
Charlson score*							
Average ± SD	5.3 ± 3.0	7.0 ± 2.2	**6.0 ± 2.8**	6.5 ± 2.0	5.4 ± 2.3	**6.0 ± 2.2**	6.0 ± 2.4
Median	5	7	**6**	7	6	**6**	6
Range	2-12	2-11	**2-12**	2-11	2-10	**2-11**	2-12
Charlson score category**							
Low (0 to 3)	10 (38.5%)	1 (5.9%)	**11 (25.6%)**	4 (8.3%)	10 (25.6%)	**14 (16.1%)**	25 (19.2%)
Moderate (4,5)	5 (19.2%)	2 (11.8%)	**7 (16.3%)**	7 (14.6%)	9 (23.1%)	**16 (18.4%)**	23 (17.7%)
High (6,7)	5 (19.2%)	7 (41.2%)	**12 (27.9%)**	24 (50%)	14 (35.9%)	**38 (43.7%)**	50 (38.5%)
Very high (8 and above)	6 (23.1%)	7 (41.2%)	**13 (30.2%)**	13 (27.1%)	6 (15.4%)	**19 (21.8%)**	32 (24.6%)

(*$p=0.0152$, ANOVA on the 4 modalities; $p=0.9435$, Student t-test comparing PD to HD patients; **$p=0.0061$, Chi Square on the 4 modalities (mild+moderate *vs.* high+very high); $p=0.8243$, Chi Square comparing PD with HD).

Most patients remained on dialysis for the entire study period; however sixteen (12.3%, 7 on PD and 9 on HD; $p=0.6651$) patients died during the 1-year study period and five (all in the HD group) patients received a kidney transplantation.

The average time on dialysis during the study was 11.1±4.9 months for HD and 10.7±6.7 months for PD (p=0.3496).

Medical Resource Use

Results on resource use are shown in Table **4**. PD patients were hospitalized on average 1.7 ± 2.0 times during the study period compared with 1.4 ± 1.6 times for HD patients (p=0.3620). PD patients spent overall an average of 19.1 ± 28.6 days in hospital (annual rate) and HD patients 17.6 ± 29.5 days (p=0.7712). The most important reason for hospitalization in the PD group was peritonitis (16.4%). Overall, 18 peritonitis episodes were observed in 13 patients (12 hospitalizations in 11 patients). The peritonitis rate was 0.45 per patient-year. In the HD group, the most important reason for hospitalization was related to the vascular access (21.3%). A further 4 hospitalizations (3.3%) were observed for access-site infections. Other reasons for hospitalization worth mentioning include bacteremia/sepsis (2.5% of HD and 1.4% of PD hospitalizations), pneumonia/bronchitis (2.5% of HD and 5.5% of PD hospitalizations), and fall (5.7% of HD and 1.4% of PD hospitalizations). Ambulatory care included laboratory tests, imaging techniques, clinic visits, interventions and medications. More ambulatory laboratory tests were performed in the HD group (295.6±137.7 *vs.* 120.1±75.5; p<0.0001). No differences were observed for imaging tests (p=0.4550). Ambulatory medications were used more frequently by HD patients (p=0.0254). The type of medications varied a lot, but the most frequently used were vitamins (Vit D - 81% of the patients), calcium (79%), erythropoiesis stimulating agents (79%), iron (59%), diuretics (55%), antihypertensive drugs (55%), H2-blockers/proton pump-inhibitors (42%), analgesics (36%), sedatives/anxiolytics (32%) and antibiotics (27%). Interventions and outpatients visits were more frequently performed in the PD group (p=0.0042), the latter being related to the pattern of care in PD patients (*i.e.*, seeing the nephrologist at the outpatient clinic rather than at the dialysis unit for HD patients).

Transport

PD patients most often used private means of transport (97.7%) to go to the hospital, *i.e.*, for dialysis purpose or for an outpatient visit. In contrast, HD patients used private transport in only 16% of cases. Most HD patients (66.7%) used "other means of transport" to go to the hospital, which was in most cases transport organized by the sickness-fund or the hospital (Table **4**).

Table 4: Medical/non-medical resource use.

	APD N=26	CAPD N=17	All PD N=43	ICHD N=48	LCHD N=39	All HD N=87	All patients N=130	P value (PD vs. HD)
Number of days in hospital (± SD)	12.9 ± 20.2	28.7 ± 36.3	**19.1 ± 28.6**	27.8 ± 36.3	4.9 ± 6.6	**17.6 ± 29.5**	18.1 ± 29.1	0.7711
Hospitalization rate (± SD)	1.4 ± 1.7	2.2 ± 2.2	**1.70 ± 2.0**	2.0 ± 1.8	0.7 ± .97	**1.40 ± 1.6**	1.5 ± 1.7	0.3620
Ambulatory care per year (number ± SD)								
Lab tests	121.0 ± 66.5	118.8 ± 89.6	**120.1 ± 75.5**	296.6 ± 157.3	294.4 ± 110.9	**295.6 ± 137.7**	237.6 ± 146.1	<0.0001
Imaging tests	5.1 ± 4.8	5.2 ± 6.6	**5.1 ± 5.5**	7.0 ± 5.1	4.3 ± 3.4	**5.8 ± 4.6**	5.6 ± 4.9	0.4550
Ambulatory consultations	7.8 ± 4.6	12.5 ± 12.5	**9.7 ± 8.8**	4.2 ± 5.7	5.2 ± 11.8	**4.6 ± 8.9**	6.3 ± 9.2	0.0029
Ambulatory interventions	3.8 ± 4.9	8.9 ± 16.3	**5.8 ± 11.1**	0.8 ± 1.3	0.5 ± 0.9	**0.7 ± 1.1**	2.4 ± 6.8	0.0042
Medications	10.4 ± 4.5	11.2 ± 4.1	**10.7 ± 4.3**	13.0 ± 3.7	11.7 ± 3.8	**12.4 ± 3.7**	11.8 ± 4.0	0.0254
% receiving EPO	73.1	88.2	**79.1**	83.3	74.4	**79.3**	79.2	
Average EPO dose†	10 488 ± 10 266	9 547 ± 10 176	**12 794 ± 10 119**	13 748 ± 18 951	8 116 ± 10 000	**11 223 ± 15 761**	10 857 ± 14 114	0.6295
Transport type used to go to hospital (for dialysis or visits)*								
Ambulance	0%	0%	**0%**	2.1%	0%	**1.1%**	0.8%	
Taxi	0%	0%	**0%**	27.1%	0%	**14.9%**	10.0%	
Private car	100.0%[§]	94.1%[¶]	**97.7%**	6.3%	28.2%	**16.1%**	43.1%	
Public transport	0%	0%	**0%**	2.1%	0%	**1.1%**	0.8%	
Other	11.5%	11.8%	**11.6%**	62.5%	71.8%	**66.7%**	48.5%	

*<0.0001 Chi Square on PD *vs.* HD; [§] 2 patients used private transport 65-75% of time and another transport the rest of time; 1 patient used private transport 37% of time and another transport for the rest of time; [¶] 1 patient used private transport 69% of time and another transport the rest of time).

Observed Costs

The observed annual costs for the different dialysis modalities are shown in Table 5. The observed cost to the MoSA was €55,296 per annum for a PD patient and €66,926 for a HD patient (p=0.0020).

Table 5: Observed costs.

	APD N=26	CAPD N=17	PD N=43	ICHD N=48	LCHD N=39	HD N=87	All patients N=130	p value (PD vs. HD)
Total	51,271 ± 13,592	61,451 ± 16,380	**55,296 ± 15,412**	80,338 ± 28,252	50,420 ± 9.957	**66,926 ± 26,541**	63,079 ± 24,024	0.0020
Dialysis procedure	*37, 916 ± 9,661*	*37,219 ± 7,018*	***37, 641 ± 8,627***	*51,790 ± 13,178*	*36,507 ± 7,750*	***44, 939 ± 13,412***	*42, 525 ± 12,492*	0.0002
Other medical and non-medical costs	*13,355 ± 13,364*	*24,232 ± 18,567*	***17, 655 ± 16,327***	*28, 548 ± 30,188*	*13,913 ± 10,800*	***21, 987± 24,559***	*20, 554 ± 22,206*	0.2343
Hospital	6,097 ± 9,248	14,612 ± 17,364	**9,463 ± 13,546**	15,338 ± 20,954	3,421 ± 6,458	**9,996 ± 21,237**	9,820 ± 18,987	0.8627
Ambulatory care	7,191 ± 7,820	9,578 ± 7,072	**8,135 ± 7,539**	12,532 ± 9,578	9,761 ± 8,358	**11,290 ± 9130**	10,247 ± 8,735	0.0523
Transport	67 ± 82	41 ± 47	**57 ± 71**	677 ± 589	731 ± 618	**701 ± 599**	488 ± 758	<0.0001

Average Cost Per Dialysis Patient in Belgium

These observed costs were multiplied by the proportion of use of the different dialysis modalities in 2006 in Belgium (*i.e.*, 6 % APD, 4% CAPD, 66% ICHD and 24% LCHD) to obtain the average cost per dialysis patient. The average annual cost of a dialysis patient to the Belgian MoSA was estimated at €70,649±€19,893 (Fig. 1). The dialysis procedure was the main cost driver (66% of costs) followed by hospitalization and ambulatory services (each 16%) while the non-medical (*i.e.*, transport) represented only 1% of the costs to the MoSA. The average annual cost of a PD patient was 31% lower than for a HD patient (€55,343±€5,080 *vs.* €72,350±€19,959 for HD). The dialysis procedure *per se* was 27% more expensive for HD, while hospital and ambulatory services were respectively 28% and 45% more expensive for HD than PD patients.

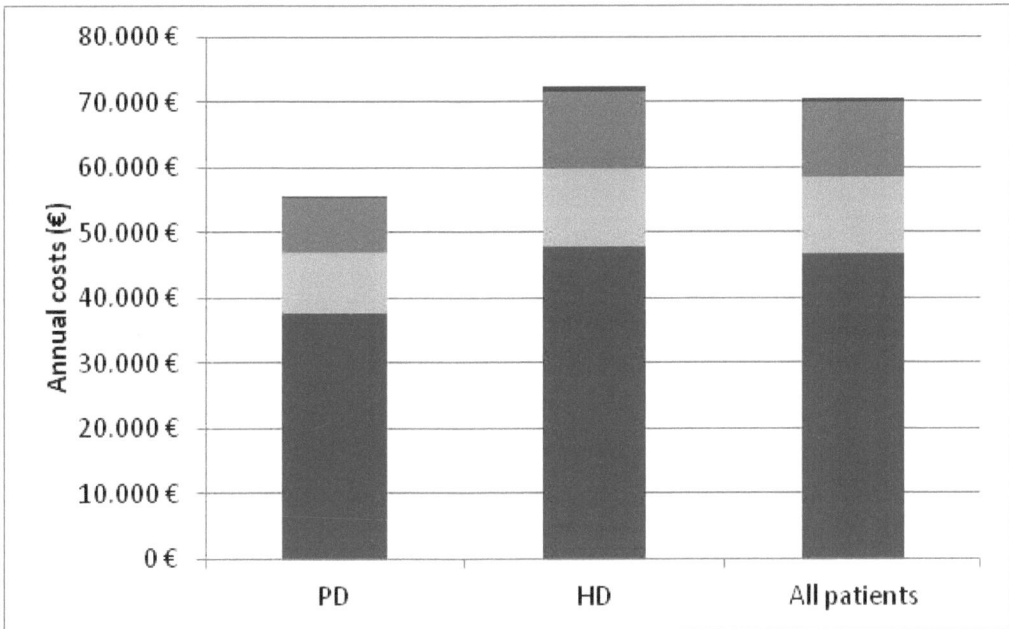

Figure 1: Average costs of a dialysis patient in Belgium (based on current usage of ICHD, LCHD, APD and CAPD) p value (HD *vs.* PD) <0.0001.

■Dialysis procedure   ▦Hospital care   ▩Ambulatory care   ■Transport

Factors Influencing the Costs

A multivariate regression showed that the 3 variables tested (dialysis technique, gender and CCI-score category) had all a significant influence on the costs of dialysis patients. The costs were 16.3% higher for HD patients (p=0.0039) and 13% lower in men than in women (p=0.0207). Furthermore, the costs of patients with a low or moderate CCI-score were respectively 21.1% and 21.0% lower than those with a very high score (p=0.0072 and p=0.0094 respectively). The costs of patients with a very high CCI-score were 10.7% higher than the costs of those with a high score, but this difference did not reach statistical significance (p=0.1160).

Estimation of the Annual Economic Burden to the MoSA

The average cost per dialysis patient (*i.e.*, €70,649) was multiplied by the total number of patients on dialysis in 2006 (*i.e.*, 6607) to obtain the economic burden of dialysis patients, *i.e.*, approximately €467 million.

DISCUSSION AND CONCLUSIONS

A retrospective review of patient records was used to estimate the economic burden of dialysis patients to the Belgian public healthcare payer. This study confirms that HD is more expensive than PD to the Belgian public healthcare payer, whether the dialysis procedure only is considered or a broader perspective (including costs of hospitalizations, ambulatory care, transport and patient costs) is taken. This study also shows that hospitalizations and ambulatory care represent a significant proportion (16% each or 32%) of the healthcare costs of dialysis patients. The annual costs of a HD patient to the Belgian healthcare system have been estimated to €72,350 (with the current usage of ICHD/LCHD). In comparison, PD patient costs were estimated at €55,343 (considering the current usage of CAPD and APD). The total annual cost of a HD patient to the MoSA in Belgium is thus 31% higher than for a PD patient. The dialysis procedure *per se* is 27% more expensive, while hospitalization and ambulatory care are 28% and 45% more expensive respectively.

As for any study, this study has some limitations. The first one is that the cost estimations are based on a sample of 130 dialysis patients. The planned randomization strategy did not work and the number of patients in the PD group (n=43) was lower than that of the HD group (n=87). Nonetheless, the PD patient sample represented 6.5% of the total Belgian PD population in 2006 (43/656). In comparison, the HD patient sample represented 1.4% of the total HD population (87/6,173). Thus, although one could argue that too few PD patients were included in the study, compared with the Belgian dialysis population, the PD patient sample represents a larger proportion.

The second limitation is that although using the official MoSA tariffs is appropriate for assessing the costs to the MoSA, it says nothing about the appropriateness of the MoSA tariffs. In Belgium, tariffs are negotiated between the INAMI/RIZIV and the healthcare providers. The dialysis tariffs have been last negotiated in 2003. However, supply costs are likely to have changed since then and this might results in disproportionate losses or profits to the supplier. Furthermore, using the MoSA perspective can significantly underestimate the overall economic burden of a disease if a large portion of the costs is paid by the patient or a third party. This is not the case for dialysis in Belgium however as dialysis patients are exempted from co-payment on the dialysis procedure, which represents 66% of the costs. The only exception is transport costs, for which the MoSA covers only about a third; hence, the MoSA perspective significantly underestimates the economic burden of transport costs.

Some may suggest that the study should have been limited to the dialysis procedure and dialysis-related healthcare costs such as dialysis access or transport. However, this would not give the full picture of the economic burden of dialysis patients to the MoSA. Quinn *et al.,* (2011) have shown that patients on dialysis tend to be hospitalized for longer period of time than patients that do not undergo dialysis, irrespective of the reason for hospitalization.

The CCI-score was used as an attempt to control for differences in health status between modalities. Although this index was not derived from End Stage Renal Disease (ESRD) patients, it remains widely used in observational research in this population (Seliger, 2010). Other indexes have been derived from small samples of ESRD patients, but have not been shown to perform substantially better than the CCI (Seliger, 2010).

Another limitation might be the center and patient selection. The centers were to be selected based on their geographical location (North, South, and Brussels) and hospital characteristics (university or university character, community hospital). Nine Belgian dialysis centers accepted to participate: all non-university centers (5 of them however with a university character) and 2 of them were linked to each other (head dialysis centre (providing only HD), satellite center (providing only PD). Geographical distribution of the centers was successful (4 North, 3 South, 2 Brussels). There is always a chance that the medical practice of the participating centers is not representative of the medical practice in Belgium. However, these 9 centers accounted for about 15% of the total number of dialysis centers in Belgium (61) (EPD, 2006-2007) and they care for 16.6% (1,138/6,829) of the total number of Belgian patients on dialysis.

Record review, as used in this study, is dependent on the quality of record keeping. Missing data will consequently lead to underestimation of the real costs.

This means however that the reported costs are conservative and that the real burden can only be higher. The same approach has been used for the two different dialysis techniques, and thus the same underestimation is expected to be seen in the 2 arms. Therefore, the relative differences between the arms are probably correct.

Indirect costs (*i.e.*, patient and caregiver time lost from work or leisure) were not captured in the study. HD patients need to go to the hospital 3 times a week for about 4-6 hours (including recovery and transport) while PD patients require 1-2 hours per day to do the exchanges. We assumed that 50% of PD patients would obtain paid help and thus the higher PD tariff for assisted-PD was used in this proportion in the calculation. This increases the costs to the public payer, but reduces the burden to patients and caregivers. Adding indirect costs is likely to widen the difference between HD and PD. Van Biesen, Lameire, Peeters and Vanholder (2007) reported the 2001 annual expenditure of a sample of 36 HD and PD patients in one Belgian university based hospital to be €78,000 for ICHD, €55,000 for LCHD and €45,000 for PD. Inflated to 2007 using an actualization factor of 1.11computed from the 2001 and 2007 health indexes (NIS, 2007) this would give €86,580 for ICHD, €61,050 for LCHD and €49,950 for PD. It is difficult to compare our findings (multi-center study) with the results from 1 center (university hospital), especially that reimbursement of dialysis has changed in 2001. Nonetheless, this study is additional evidence that HD is more expensive than PD as shown by several national/international studies and reviews (Benain *et al.*, 2007; Berger, Edelsberg, Inglese, Bhattacharyya, & Oster, 2009; Gheyle, Jeggers, & Matthijs, 1994; Lee *et al.*, 2002; Peeters, Rublee, Just, & Joseph, 2000). A lot of these studies however, focused on the procedure costs only.

A recent Belgian report of the Federal Knowledge Centre (KCE) focusing on the organization and financing of chronic dialysis in Belgium (Cleemput *et al.*, 2010) reported costs for the different dialysis methods from the public health care payer perspective were comparable to our own findings.

Assuming that the dialysis costs calculated in our study are representative for Belgium, and taking into account that at the end of 2006, about 6,607 patients (0.06% of the Belgian population) were on dialysis, the total cost of dialysis for the MoSA would have been 467 million Euro (very close to the official figure of 450 million Euro reported by the KCE). This represents 2.45% of the 18.43-billion healthcare budget (Belgium Chamber of Representatives, 2008).

Therefore, increasing PD use from the current 10% to 30% could generate savings to the MoSA in the order of €22 million per year. Hence, this would allow treating about 325 additional patients with the same budget.

In conclusion, our study shows that for a group of patients with similar levels of co-morbidity, the total costs (*i.e.*, including ambulatory care and hospitalization in addition to the dialysis procedure costs) are higher for HD than PD patients and that important savings to the healthcare system could be expected not only from the procedure costs but also from other medical and non-medical costs by using PD in more patients.

ACKNOWLEDGEMENT

None Declared.

CONFLICT OF INTEREST

None Declared.

REFERENCES

Beddhu S, Burns FJ, Saul M, Seddon P, Zeidel ML. (2000). A simple comorbidity scale predicts clinical outcomes and costs in dialysis patients. Am J Med, 108, 609-613.

Belgium Chamber of Representatives (2008) Belgische Kamer van Volksvertegenwoordigers/Chambre des Representants de Belgique, Voorstel van Resolutie/ Proposition de Resolution DOC: 52 0687/001. 16 January 2008. Retrieved from: http://www.lachambre.be/FLWB/PDF/52/0687/52K0687001.pdf.

Benain JP, Faller B, Briat C, Jacquelinet C, Brami M, Aoustin M *et al.* (2007). Cost of dialysis in France. Nephrol Ther, 3(3), 96-106.

Berger A, Edelsberg J, Inglese GW, Bhattacharyya SK, Oster G. (2009). Cost comparison of peritoneal dialysis *versus* hemodialysis in end-stage renal disease. Am J Manag Care, 15(8):509-18.

Cleemput I, Beguin C, La Kethulle, Gerkens S, Jadoul M, Verpooten G *et al.* (2010). Organisation et Financement de la Dialyse Chronique en Belgique. KCE report 124A, Retrieved July 5, 2012 from: https://kce.fgov.be/sites/default/files/page_documents/d20101027312.pdf

EPD (2006-2007) European Practice Database, Report Belgium. Retrieved from http://www.orpadt.be/documenten/EPDResultsFlandersWallonia2007.pdf

ERA-EDTA Registry. (2009). ERA-EDTA Registry Annual report 2007. Academic Medical Center, Department of Medical Informatics, Amsterdam, The Netherlands. Retrieved July 5, 2012, from: http://www.era-edta-reg.org/files/annualreports/pdf/AnnRep2007.pdf

ERA-EDTA Registry (2011). ERA-EDTA Registry Annual report 2009. Academic Medical Center, Department of Medical Informatics, Amsterdam, The Netherlands. Retrieved July 5, 2012 from: http://www.era-edta-reg.org/files/annualreports/pdf/AnnRep2009_new.pdf

Gheyle D, Jegers M, Matthijs P. (1994). Kostenvergelijking tussen twee vormen van nierfunctievervangende therapie: continue ambulante peritoneale dialyse en centrum hemodialyse (Comparison of costs and revenues of renal disease therapies). Tijdschrift voor Geneeskunde, 50,12.

Just PM, Riella MC, Tschosik EA, Noe LL, Bhattacharyya SK, de Charro FT. (2008). Economic Evaluations of Dialysis Treatment Modalities. Health Policy, 86, 163-180.

Kramer A, Stel V, Zoccali C, Heaf J, Ansell D, Gronhagen-Riska C *et al.* (2009). An update on renal replacement therapy in Europe: ERA-EDTA Registry data from 1997 to 2006. Nephrol Dial Transplant, 24(12), 3557-3566.

Lee H, Manns B, Taub K, Ghali WA, Stafford D, Johnson D *et al.* (2002). Cost analysis of ongoing care of patients with end-stage renal disease: the impact of dialysis modality and dialysis access. Am J Kidney Dis, 40(3), 611-622.

NIS (2007) National Institute for Statistics. Consumer price index since 1920 and health index since 1994. Retrieved from: http://statbel.fgov.be/en/statistics/figures/economy/consumer_price_index/

Peeters P, Rublee D, Just PM, Joseph A. (2000). Analysis and interpretation of cost data in dialysis: review of Western European literature. Health Policy, 54(3), 209-227.

Quinn MP, Cardwell CR, Rainey A, McNamee PT, Kee F, Maxwell AP *et al.* (2011). Patterns of hospitalization before and following initiation of haemodialysis: a 5-year single centre study. Postgrad Med J, *87*, 389-393.

INAMI/RIZIV (2007) Institut National d'assurance Maladie-Invalidité/ Rijksinstituut voor Ziekte- en Invaliditeitsverzekering 2007 tariffs. Retrieved from : http://www.inami.be/insurer/fr/rate/history/history2007.htm

Seliger SL. (2010). Comorbidity and confounding in end-stage renal disease. Kidney Int, *77*(2), 83-85.

Van Biesen W, Lameire N, Peeters P, Vanholder R. Belgium's mixed private/public health care system and its impact on the cost of end-stage renal disease. (2007). Int J Health Care Finance Econ, 7(2-3), 133-148.

Send Orders of Reprints at reprints@benthamscience.net

CHAPTER 13

Conclusion - Use of Patient Reported Outcomes Measures by the Pharmaceutical Industry

Paraskevi Theofilou[1,2,*]

[1]*Sotiria Hospital for Thoracic Diseases, Athens, Greece and* [2]*Center for Research and Technology, Department of Kinesiology, Health & Quality of Life Research Group, Trikala, Thessaly, Greece*

INTRODUCTION

Health care outcomes research came into fashion in the early 1980s, as the more academic counterpart to health policy research (Matchar & Rudd, 2005). Measurement of quality of life was considered a key factor and a catalytic element in the implementation of outcomes management (Ellwood, 1989), making the interpretation of the results of these measurements a crucial step in the implementation process.

Ellwood (1988) suggested that physicians could use outcomes management to bring a better quality of life to their patients, implying that quality of life itself is an outcome that must be measured to better gauge the success of outcomes management.

As a result, the pharmaceutical research community recognized the value of measuring quality of life outcomes during drug development.

In light of developments such as these, standardized patient - report measures for evaluating treatment impact were increasingly introduced in clinical trials for new drug development, including multi item quality of life or general health measures. The first major medical journal report of a clinical trial in which health - related quality of life was used as a primary endpoint (Croog *et al.*, 1986) - albeit capturing tolerability more than efficacy - not only generated a surge of activity

Address correspondence to Paraskevi Theofilou: Sotiria Hospital for Thoracic Diseases, Athens, Greece; Center for Research and Technology, Department of Kinesiology, Health & Quality of Life Research Group, Trikala, Thessaly, Greece; Tel: +0030 6977441502, Fax: +0030 2106221435; E-mail: theofi@otenet.gr; paraskevi.theofilou@gmail.com

within the pharmaceutical industry to include similar outcome measures in clinical studies to support new drug approval or provide them with product differentiation by using quality of life claims in promotional materials, but also had an economic impact (Bishop, 1986).

Industry - sponsored patient related outcomes (PRO) use cores mainly around inclusion in clinical medicine and patient registries. Nowadays, PRO endpoints are used in a few clinical trials. However, their use is extensive recently, principally in randomized Phase III trials.

The main question which arises is "Does the industry use these PRO data?" It is well known that companies need a PRO policy for an innovative complex in order to consider all likely means of making attracted parties aware of relevant information. Also, communication is a matter of great importance. Specifically, if a company wants to keep track with developments in rising methods of communication, strategies for distribution of key messages will need to advance. It is essential for the industries to know that the most excellent use of PRO data presupposes distribution of them as extensively as possible to all key stakeholders. Unfortunately, despite the growing use of PRO endpoints in clinical medicine and patient registries, a large number of the data collected remains underutilized and frequently unreported (Doward, Gnanasakthy & Baker, 2010). Whether or not a successful PRO - based label claim is achieved, PRO data collected for research purposes should be published in scientific journals. Another attitude which characterizes the industry is that it casts aside PRO data as unworthy of further attention. This happens because too often they are considered unsuitable for a label claim by authorities. On the other side, researchers, in order to conduct secondary analyses or even prepare a paper to be published in a scientific journal, frequently find it difficult to give explanation for the resources needed. However, key stakeholders show much interest in PRO - evidence. As clinicians particularly become more doubtful regarding conventional sales methods, academic publications become the answer for presenting product value messages (Price water house Coppers, 2009). Yet, knowledge included in research publications has always been available only for those specialists who are fortunate enough to have the chance working in a university that subscribes to specific journals. On the other hand, we should accept the fact that the availability of rising technologies has effectively broadened the audience able to enter to the scientific information (Doward *et al.*, 2010). Particularly, patients are very interested in identifying information on those treatment benefits that are of interest to them - and even more interested in distributing useful findings *via* websites. Additionally to providing data concerning treatment effectiveness, secondary analysis can be conducted on PRO data collected in the context of clinical trials to provide disease or drug intelligence. An investigation of the key demographic (age, gender, education, marital status, work status *etc.*), psychological (depression, anxiety, health locus of control *etc.*) as well as clinical variables (duration, severity, diagnostic groupings *etc.*) influencing for example, patient perceived severity of condition, health - related quality of life or functional status can further our understanding of the disease from the patient's point of view (Stull *et al.*, 2009). This can provide an examination of predictors of functional status and quality of life impact, information on mediating factors in disease severity and implications for treatment, especially product targeting (Doward *et al.*, 2010). Secondary analysis can provide market intelligence in an effective way and with a reduced cost that can be fed into company strategies for targeted drug development and marketing (Doward *et al.*, 2010). Again, it is essential to indicate that the distribution of such information *via* the publications in scientific journals as well as the support of this distribution *via* web-based technologies must be fully encouraged. The company's commitment to patients as well as its reputation with patient groups and clinicians is an important matter. The solution for this achievement is the presentation of well thought out PRO - based information, whether this relates to product usefulness or disease intelligence.

ACKNOWLEDGEMENT

None Declared.

CONFLICT OF INTEREST

None Declared.

REFERENCES

Bishop J. (1986). Squibb drug called superior in easing high blood pressure: findings of medical journal are leaked, prompting a jump in price of stock. Wall Street Journal (6/25).

Croog SH, Levine S, Testa MA, Brown B, Bulpitt CJ, Jenkins CD, *et al.* (1986). The effects of antihypertensive therapy on the quality of life. N Engl J Med, 314(26): 1657-64.

Doward CL, Gnanasakthy A, Baker GM. (2010). Patient reported outcomes: looking beyond the label claim Health and Quality of Life Outcomes, 8:89 1-9.

Ellwood PM. (1988). Shattuck Lecture - Outcomes management: a technology of patient experience. N Engl J Med, 318(23):1549-56.

Ellwood PM. (1989). Outcomes management: new name for old idea. Interview by Wesley Curry. Physician Exec, 15(5):2-6.

Matchar DB, Rudd AG. (2005). Health policy and outcomes research 2004. Stroke, 36(2): 225-227.

PricewaterhouseCoppers. Pharma 2020. (2009). Marketing the future. Which path will you take. PricewaterhouseCoopers.

Stull D, Wyrwich KW, Frueh FW. (2009). Methods for personalised medicine: Factor mixture models for investigating differential response to treatment. Value Health, 12(3): A27.

INDEX

A

Abate dialysis 48

Adherence behaviours 114, 117, 119-20, 126, 129

Adherence interventions 130, 138

Adherence levels 121-2, 128-9, 147

Adherence questionnaire 124-5

Adherence rates 7, 112-13, 118, 128, 131

Adherence to treatment and interventions 7

Adolescent renal transplant patients 85, 87

Advanced chronic kidney disease 80, 87

Aerobic exercise 40

African-American caregivers of dialysis patients 173

Albumin 52, 143, 145, 147, 149

Anxiety 4-5, 28, 30, 38, 102-3, 167, 170, 173-6, 193, 225

Anxiety/depression 30, 127

Anxiety disorders 54

APD and CAPD patients 63

Applications of QoL research 6, 47-8

Audit of diabetes dependent quality of Life (ADDQoL) 33

Automatic peritoneal dialysis (APD) 63, 114, 116, 210-12, 216-18

B

BDI scores in CAPD patients 63

Behavioral interventions 138, 140

Benton visual retention test (BVRT) 101

Bicarbonate 205-6

Bicarbonate cartridge 200

Bicarbonate dialysis 8, 198

Bicarbonate dialysis program 202

Bicarbonate solution 200, 202, 205

Biochemical markers 52, 98, 112, 119-20, 131

Blood urea nitrogen (BUN) 120, 125, 143, 147, 149-50